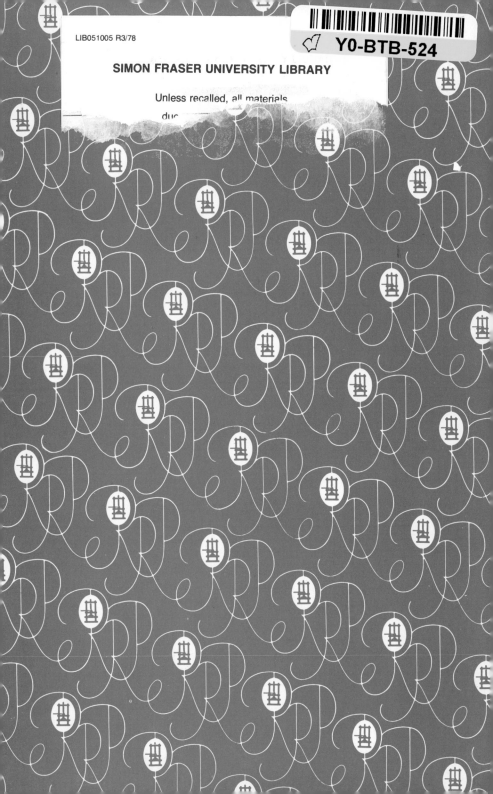

ENJOYING THE ARTS/DANCE

ENJOYING THE ARTS

Dance

By

Nancy Meadors Kline

Illustrated by

Laura Eynon

RICHARDS ROSEN PRESS, INC.
New York, N.Y. 10010

Published in 1975 by Richards Rosen Press, Inc.
29 East 21st Street, New York, N.Y. 10010

First Edition

Library of Congress Cataloging in Publication Data

Kline, Nancy Meadors.
   Enjoying the arts: dance.

   SUMMARY: Presents a background of modern dance
and ballet, introduces such innovators as Martha Graham,
Isadora Duncan, and José Límon, and discusses such works
as "Petrouchka" and "Appalachian Spring."
   1. Dancing. [1. Dancing] I. Eynon, Laura, illus.
II. Title.
GV1593.K57   793.3′2   73–91271
ISBN 0–8239–0296–X

Manufactured in the United States of America

TO MOTHER AND DAD
Who gave me dance lessons
instead of the red boots

ABOUT THE AUTHOR
AND ILLUSTRATOR

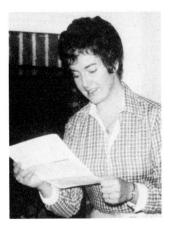 NANCY MEADORS KLINE is currently the director and co-teacher of The Interlocking Curriculum at Sandy Spring Friends School, Sandy Spring, Maryland. She and her husband, Peter Kline, have created a one-year curriculum for high-school students that increases motivation and capacity to learn. Many of these courses Nancy Kline developed, her favorite being a poetry and dance course that helps students explore and enjoy poetry by experiencing it first through body movement. Dance has always been a major part of her teaching and of her personal life. She has found that students who learn to express ideas and images through dance understand those ideas better. While her students learn to use dance in this way, they also grow to appreciate and understand the masterpieces discussed in her book. The combination contributes to a rich and exciting curriculum.

Nancy Kline received a Bachelor of Arts degree in 1968 from Scripps College, Claremont, California. There she concentrated in literature and dance. She has taught for five years, two of them at The Madeira School in Virginia. She also is a consultant for Mankind Research Unlimited, Inc. Her other publications include *Physical Movement for the Theater* and "Scientist in a Strange Land," published by Potomac Magazine.

About the Author and Illustrator

LAURA EYNON, the illustrator, is a student of art and aesthetics at Sandy Spring Friends School in Sandy Spring, Maryland. She is currently studying the relationships between dance and drawing and is concentrating on the potential for abstraction in the human form.

CONTENTS

Contents

ACKNOWLEDGMENTS

I wish to thank the following persons who helped make this book possible:

Edelweiss Meadors for her invaluable and expert editing of the manuscript, and for her loving and dependable impressions of the West;

Dianne McLean for her efficient and beautiful job as typist of the manuscript;

Glee Collins for the use of her treasured photographs and etchings of early dancers;

Marna Lucychyn and Henry Wisneski of the staff of the Dance Collection, New York City Public Library for the Performing Arts;

Rebecca Cooprider for her sensitive comments on an early draft;

Jean Parker Smith for the present time this book reflects;

Katherine Wiborg, who was an important part of every dance I ever created;

Beatrice Richardson for Orchesis and June programs and wisdom;

and Peter Kline, who knew I would do this long before I did.

LIST OF ILLUSTRATIONS

INTRODUCTION

Dance cannot be read. It cannot faithfully be written about. To be truly understood, it must be danced. This book, therefore, is meant only as a companion to your real dance experience. It cannot replace the visceral knowledge that dance re-creates profound human emotions; you will know that when you have done it. But as you are learning about dance by dancing, this book can provide an intellectual appreciation of the movements your body must someday execute; it can create in you an awareness of the human lives behind the dances you will be seeing at the theatre; and it can offer a point of view of parts of those dances to enlarge your movement vocabulary and to make clearer how the choreographer chose the movement-words she did to express her ideas.

The irony of any discussion of dance is that it requires us to stop in time a medium that at its very essence is time-moving. It is more true of dance than anything else that to focus on one part of a piece is to lose its meaning, since its existence depends upon what went before it and what will follow. But we will do this impossible thing with the realization that whatever we say together is miles away from the dance itself and with the purpose that when the dance is actually experienced, this discussion will have enriched our receptivity to it.

To this end, we will look at what movement is, at how it defines our very existence. We will see how movement got itself structured from random activity into dance, looking first at dance called ballet and then at modern dance. We will look at five human experiences and how they are re-created in specific moments of five ballets and five modern dance compositions. We also will get well acquainted with two people who are dancing today and who will add new slants to the ideas and impressions we have experienced in reading this book.

The book is unique because it produces a flavor toward dance as it elicits from you a feeling for what dance can do. Fuller histories, more documented accounts, larger volumes on dance are available, and these should be read and enjoyed also. But this book is intended as an excursion that should be made on a breezy day with all imaginative gears unlocked. It is intended equally for the student who thinks of dance as something his snarly little sisters did after school on Tuesdays, for those who have season tickets each year to the ballet and long for the return of the Bolshoi, and for those who trace their first sense of honesty in themselves to their first modern dance composition. It is a placement of dance in life as we know it without removing it from its special place as art.

Hopefully, you will someday see some of the dances you will read about here. Hopefully, you will enjoy them immensely as you recognize, agree with, and take issue with the things we have said about them. Perhaps, too, you will someday create your own dances and truly know dance for the first time. But, regardless, you will see life differently—you will no longer miss the movements all around you; you will recognize them in design as bricks climb the side of a building, in sound as bells join tubas and strings and kettledrums, and in bodies whether as capsulized life onstage or as you are caught in a sticky moment having heard somewhere that movement never lies. Out of this movement comes dance, the truest, deepest form of human expression.

PART ONE

I

NOTHING IS EVER STILL

Atoms move. Insides of atoms move. The tiniest known particle is nothing but motion. If atoms and molecules are motion, then cells and tissues, muscles, bodies, hair, sweat, chairs, rugs, basements, watermelons are motion. There is no such thing as something solid. Everything, except empty space, is movement. If a rotten lemon is softer than a bathtub, it is because the clumps of motion are less tightly packed. There is more empty space between them. But when you get right down to it, all we are is movement. Nothing is ever still.

*   *   *

"Daddy, won't you take me back to Muleinberg County? Down by the blue rivers where paradise lay?"
"I'm sorry my son, but you're too late in askin'. Mr. Peabody's coal train has hauled it away."

John Prine

*   *   *

"The Tigre primitives dance the chassé step in a circle. They keep time by shrugging their shoulders and moving their elbows backward and forward. Periodically the dancers squat on the ground; they continue to move their arms and shoulders in this way."

*   *   *

All quotations in this chapter, unless otherwise designated, are from Lincoln Kirstein, *Dance: A Short History of Classic Theatrical Dancing* (New York, Dance Horizons, 1969).

3

The sea plays on and on
White waves to wash upon white waves

*   *   *

The Hopi Snake Dance begins at dawn on the mesa. Only the men of the tribe participate, and of them only those of high position. of the day, waiting until each member of the dance has purified him- They sit below the earth in the kiva (ceremonial structure) for most self and is acceptable to the gods. Finally, with no warning, they emerge with live rattlesnakes between their teeth. They move in a circle to a steady rhythmic beat that resounds across the mesa. Different patterns form, arms move toward the heavens, heads bow to the earth. When it is over, the snakes run free to take the message to the gods.

*   *   *

The mountain quivered and at its feet the thatched shacks made no notice. As it swayed and rumbled men dashed from the dried cornstalks into their homes, and waited. The mountain burst and the corn turned bronze and the shacks dissolved and became liquid.

*   *   *

"In Egypt the goddess Hathor presided over the dance. Pharaoh, as son of Hathor, is seen jingling a sistrum (ancient percussion instrument) before her, while her priests are dancing and clattering castanets. At all her festivals dancing was an indispensable feature. Afterward the priestesses and the male priests marched in the streets and stopped at the houses of the people bestowing Hathor's blessing by dancing and holding the necklace of the goddess to be touched for fertility."

*   *   *

Listen, Sissy, can you hear it?
Shhh, mommy will hear us.
Oh, come on, see if you can hear it.
I can't hear anything; but let's say I could; what do you say it is out there?
I know what it is, it's the corn growin' and tomorrow you'll be able to tell it, too.
Corn growin', huh? Gosh. I sure hope mama didn't hear that.

*   *   *

"All Greek dancing developed from the communal form of choral dance. There may have been solo dancing and *pas de deux*, but if so, they were secondary. Most frequently, the *choros* would move cyclically or circularly in its orchestra or dancing floor, but there were also the theatrical *choros*, which marched in rectangular ranks or files."

*   *   *

Your cells die and replace themselves at the rate of three billion every minute.

*   *   *

"From the Old Testament itself we have the sacred processional of King David and all the house of Israel dancing before Jehovah with all their might. In the Hebrew they are said to 'rotate with-all-their-might,' 'to jump,' 'whirl around,' and 'skip.' In the last two psalms of David, the prophet exhorts his people to 'praise His name in the dance,' 'praise him with the timbrel and the dance'."

*   *   *

From night to dawn to next year. I grow old as you grow up. But I have never been here before either.

*   *   *

5

In 604 the Christian Church danced. "In certain Paris churches the senior canon led choirboys in a round dance during the singing of the psalm. The Paris Liturgy reads 'The canon will dance to the first psalm.' Scaliger said the first Roman bishops led a sacred 'dance' around in church and in front of martyrs' tombs . . . we may assume that the movements were sufficiently timid or restricted to preclude either their offending the celebrants, exciting the participants, or in any real sense enriching the Missal."

*   *   *

My love, I pierce the colors in the sky
And seek to find you there and know not why.
The rain has finished with its violent blast,
Now peaks the sun. The rainbow's come at last.

*   *   *

"For the Dance of Death, the triumphal car was covered with black cloth, and was of vast size; it had skeletons and white crosses painted upon its surface, and was drawn by buffaloes, all of which were totally black; within the car stood the colossal figure of Death, bearing the scythe in his hand; while around him were covered tombs. At a certain distance appeared figures bearing torches, and wearing masks presenting the face of a death's head both before and behind. At the sound of a wailing summons, sent forth with a hollow moan from trumpets of muffled yet inexorable clangor, the figures of the dead raised themselves half out of their tombs, and seating their skeleton forms thereon, they sang the music of the most plaintive and melancholy character. Before and after the car rode a train of the dead on horses, four attendants bearing black torches and a large black standard. While this train proceeded each sang with a trembling voice."

*   *   *

6

Nothing Is Ever Still

I remember hearing guns and racing down the street to find Jennifer no one was there that I knew and everyone looked different all the lines in their faces were new they hadn't known anything like this before except maybe in some frantic dream but even then you can wake up and decide whether or not to let it happen again by going back to sleep that is there you couldn't decide anything it all just kept on happening I rushed toward her but everything all around me was different.

* * *

Observe said anthill. As heretofore mentioned and stated, said ants, propelled in accordance with the terms and conditions of unseen ant legs, do move and proceed to the aforesaid mound on the day and year first above mentioned when and as soon as hunting efforts, the likes of which never could be performed in like manner by man thereon, are completed, trampling by tennis shoes not withstanding. All members of said ant colony are thereby pronounced by and between ourselves as workers not surpassed by any beast heretofore known.

* * *

"The Italian dancers, for instance, wear bells, they often fight a mock-battle. The Cupids brandishing their torches, Vulcan and his Cyclops beating time with their hammers, are not so very far removed, after all, from the villagers beating time with their sticks."

* * *

Behold, the village shall stand not still. It will harbor unto itself but soon shall pass away. And, lo, I say unto you greater and greater dwellings shall come upon you. Cities of great magnitude shall you build. But hear me when I say cleave not

7

to things which come not from the earth. False objects shall your destruction be.

*   *   *

By 1600 dancing had developed into a form known as The Ballet Comique. "It was a kind of game and dance which involved three men and three ladies. The first young man would lead his damsel to the end of the room, when he would return alone to his companions. The second would do the same and so the third. The three girls were thereby left by themselves at one end of the room, the men at the other. The first then making all manner of amourous glances, pulling his hose tight and setting his shirt straight, went to claim his damsel, who refused him. Then, seeing that the young man had returned to his place, she pretended to be in despair. The two others did the same. Finally all three went to claim their respective damsels, kneeled on the ground, begged their good favor with clasped hands. The damsels fell into their arms and all danced together."

*   *   *

What is green, yellow, orange, gray; then blue, orange, gray; then grange, bellow; then grangello?

*   *   *

In 1730 ballet had found a place for itself in the opera. The dancing master had a master plan which he could follow for almost any production. It went like this: "Prologue: pastimes for the dancers representing Games and Pleasures; Gavotte for the Laughs; Rigaudon for the Pleasant; Musetee for the Priestesses; Loure for the People, Tambourin air for the same entry of Greeks and Chaconne, without Zephyrs."

*   *   *

Aquarians, you may expect trouble this week. Pay special attention to the clothes you wear. Beware if you are seen in a high wig and layers of petticoats. Lean instead toward a looser bodice and ringlettes, and high, high heels. Seek your changeable nature by Wednesday with a tight skirt falling just, just mind you, above the ankle. Saturn moves in your favor by Friday and will give you impulses toward shorter skirt, shorter hair, shorter collar. Go ahead! But on Saturday return, poor dearie, to cover the leg, cover the head with massive brims. And move slowly, ever so slowly, up, up, up. Why that, Miss Aquarian, is no skirt at all. Take no chances. Your watchwords are gingham and shawl. That is better. That is better.

*   *   *

Great reformer of the dance Jean Noverre wrote in his essay on the dance: "Let this restorer of the true dance appear, this reformer of bad taste. Children of Terpsichore, renounce over-complicated steps; abandon grimaces to study sentiments. Study how to make your gestures noble, never forget that is the life-blood of dancing; put judgement and sense into your *pas de deux*; away with those lifeless masks; take off those enormous wigs and those gigantic headdresses. Discard those stiff and cumbersome hoops. Let good taste preside over all situations."

*   *   *

At the sound of the tone the time will be:
eight thirty-two
and two seconds

*   *   *

Noverre's ideas became rigidified. In 1830, Carlo Blasis set down his formula for the ballerina to follow. "Let your body be, in

9

general, erect and perpendicular on your legs, except in certain attitudes, and especially in arabesque, when it must lean forwards or backwards according to the position you adopt. Keep it always equally poised upon your thighs. Throw your breast out and hold your waist in as much as you can. In your performance preserve continually a slight bend, and much firmness about your loins. Let your shoulders be low, your head high, and your countenance animated and expressive."

*   *   *

Mr. and Mrs. John Abraham, III,
request the pleasure of your company
at the marriage of their daughter
Jennifer Elizabeth
to
Sam Smith
tomorrow
around dusk
Give us a call if you're coming!

*   *   *

The beloved Maria Taglioni, one of the first to dance on her toes, did her part to return to the ideals of Noverre. "She glides over the flowers without bending them. In one print she bounces in high *jetés*. Such a wraith was undreamed of before. Everyone agrees upon her gliding lightness, the frail imponderable weight which slight limbs could never support except for their pact with ether. Her toes have 'pointes.' Her body is veiled diaphanously in misty muslin."

*   *   *

EXIT

*   *   *

Taglioni's principles, too, became rigid in the hands of others. Marius Petipa contributed his formula. In 1870, long enough after Taglioni's death to provide time for the development of her "pointes," he, creator of *Swan Lake* and *The Sleeping Beauty*, had this to say about how ballet should be danced: "The classical dance can be succinctly characterized by the use of beats on the points and beats of elevation. It contains the traditional, symmetrical forms of the *pas de deux*, a choreographical poem in three verses in a rigid framework, the adagio a chain of movements and *pirouettes* by the ballerina supported by the dancer; two variations, that of the ballerina and that of the dancer whose more restricted art is confined to leaps; lastly the coda, in which the dancer alternates with the ballerina in a succession of accelerated measures that mount up to the presto and end in a whirlwind of movements and dizzy complicated turns."

*   *   *

We are at two minutes, thirty seconds and counting . . .

*   *   *

In 1900 Isadora Duncan wrote: "It was the first time I had seen a palm tree growing in a temperate climate. I used to notice its leaves trembling in the early morning breeze, and from them I created in my dance that light fluttering of the arms, hands and fingers, which has been so much abused by my imitators; for they forget to go to the original source and contemplate the movements of the palm trees, to receive them inwardly before giving them outwardly."

*   *   *

No one is there. No one has been for hours. It must be nearly morning by now. Still the lights go on and on. Never missing. First green then yellow then red. Then green.

*   *   *

11

"The Modern Dance is couched in the rhythm of our time; it is broken and the body falls into angles, which are percussive segments of a circle—circular movement arrested. It is not important that you should know what a dance means on the stage. It is only important that you should be stirred. If you can write the story of your dance, it is a literary thing but not dancing."

Martha Graham

*   *   *

Tonight: partly cloudy
High: 65
Low: 58
Barometer: rising
Humidity: 55%
Sunrise: 5:30 a.m.
Sunset: 8:56 p.m.
Have a good weekend.

*   *   *

"They're all wondering about the new dance. But then, so am I. I don't have ideas exactly. There's no thinking involved in my choreography. I work alone for a couple of hours every morning in the studio. I just try things out. It's all in terms of the body, you see. I don't work through images or ideas—I work through the body. And I don't ever want a dancer to start thinking that a movement means something."

Merce Cunningham—1965

*   *   *

"*. . . nor can foot feel, being shod,*"
G. M. *Hopkins*

*   *   *

Nothing Is Ever Still

"Dance must get back to its spiritual roots. What the individual dancer feels, what she needs to say through dance, must become again the motivation behind movement."

Liz Lerman—1973

*   *   *

Nothing is ever still.

*   *   *

II

THE DANCE HAS MANY FORMS

Through all movement we see flickers of dance. In the most everyday kinds of motion there is the beginning, the root inspiration, or the skeleton of a dance. It is the choreographer's job to take movement from life experiences and build on them, transform, exaggerate or distort them to create dances out of them. A simple walk down the street, an overflowing Seven-Up, a wilting lilac all have elements that lead to dance. A simple walk down the street is not in itself a dance, but when a particular style of walking is extended in its lines, repeated several times, and combined with movements that we would never see on the street, it becomes the stuff of dance.

From random movement two kinds of dance can be built. One takes place in real time and real space. In this case the dancer is herself, performing a piece that takes place now on this stage and does not represent a place or time anywhere else. Tap dancing, jazz, ballroom, folk dancing, court dances, and some primitive rituals all belong to this group.

The other kind of dance is representational or symbolic. The dancers are supposed to be other people in a different time and a different place. They may also represent concepts or feelings separate from the people who embody them. The audience is supposed to experience the dance as a statement about life, as an expression of complex emotion, as more than a display of technical skill to be enjoyed at the moment. Classical ballet, modern ballet, and modern dance all belong to this group.

To achieve its effect, this kind of dance must manipulate time. The choreographer can make time longer or he can condense it to fit his purpose. In *Pillar of Fire,* for instance, the main character goes through months of anguish that were preceded by years of self-doubt, all in about twenty minutes. Antony Tudor has opened up the mental and emotional facets of his character by twisting and condensing time in this way.

Expanding time is another means of exploring the psyches of characters in dance. Martha Graham created a full-length dance dealing with the *instant* when Jocasta recognizes that she is the mother as well as the wife of Oedipus. For an hour characters "pursue themselves across her heart in that instant of agony." Dance, then, can capsulize thousands of moments into the tiniest time or expand an instant into an hour. This manipulation of time is an important tool in creating expressive, symbolic, representational dance.

Although it is true that classical ballet, modern ballet, and modern dance have in common the fact that they draw upon random movement and that they manage time to create their final effects, these final effects are often very different from one another. Classical ballet, for instance, follows closely the rules of movement set down by Petipa in the nineteenth century and concerns itself primarily with more superficial, fairyland themes in which people who are not quite real go about expressing feelings that are not quite profound. Often the story line will give way for a few minutes in real time to the display of technical skill by the *premier danseur* and his ballerina partner. The intended effect is to leave you enthralled and ecstatic with the pure pleasure of having experienced something beautiful.

Nineteenth-century ballet makes us take a deep breath and relax;

it makes us smile and sway a little and feel with the first burst of the strings that we have been enveloped in a world luscious and fluid. When ballets are performed by sensitive dancers they are really more than acrobatics, but we will always thrill to the incredible feats we see when these ballets provide sections for the premier danseur and prima ballerina to perform. This thrill—to the leaps that split the air, to the turns on one toe that display perfect balance and control, to the running lifts and their removal of the dancer from earthly laws—this thrill is an important part of what makes classical ballet so enjoyable.

Modern ballet and modern dance, on the other hand, seek to involve the audience in ways very different from classical pieces. Modern dances, with their departure from classical rules, their angles, broken lines, distorted rhythms, and themes that explore the psychological roots of human distress and happiness, are intended to leave us disturbed. We are asked to see ourselves naked and vulnerable; to go away shaken, to get a clearer picture of what we are as human beings.

This kind of dance, though frequently offering social comment, is primarily a personal statement. The best way to see this kind of dance performance is to clear the mind of preconceptions about what the dance *should* mean and let the dance unfold in whatever way it will; let it touch the areas of your life that surface readily without an intellectual struggle. Whatever comes to mind as the dance progresses, whatever stirs deep in the center of you is what the dance means. It will be different for each of us, but as we leave we will know that something common to all of us has been nudged, and briefly, if not profoundly, reconsidered.

What we gain from a new experience is largely determined by what we bring to it. If we see something we have never seen before we will try very hard to find elements in it that compare with things we have seen and that have had meaning for us. If we cannot readily find any similarities we will take little notice of the new experience. Experiences that leave us cold are usually those that seem to have no relationship with anything else we have ever learned. It is true of dance as well. Therefore, it is important to have as much understanding of dance as possible before attending a performance.

Such an understanding will include a recognition not just of the intent of a given dance but also of the historical setting from which that work emerged. To have lodged in a mental corner somewhere the realization that a Tudor ballet was originally a dramatic rebellion against the rules and fairylands of Petipa is to bring a greater appreciation to his work and to add to whatever personal meaning the work has for you. To keep in mind that Martha Graham was even wilder and more rebellious than Tudor in her beliefs about what dance should be is to bring to any performance of her work a kind of appreciation that is not possible otherwise.

It would be well, then, to take a few moments to see this history in action, to get an idea of how random movement grown into dance eventually found itself structured into the most stirring description of the human condition to be found anywhere.

III

BALLET TO THE PRESENT

Ballet begins with high heels. It begins with skirts puffed out with whalebone frames at the hips, towering wigs, huge feathers, and long, heavy fabrics. You need only to dress up in these eighteenth-century things, or even to imagine doing so, to realize that the dancer was not about to take off into the lyrical leaps and staccato turns and delicate arabesques that we associate with ballet. These cumbersome costumes allowed for elegant walks, gestures, and pantomime here and there, but certainly nothing we would pay $6.50 a seat for today. It was a beginning, however, and we should take a look at it for what it tells us of the dances we see today.

This early form of ballet, seen primarily in opera, was in its own way a liberation for dance. It was a step toward identifying ballet as something distinct from court celebrations, religious rites, and processions. We laugh to think of dressing in toe shoes and pirouetting into a neighborhood party, but there was a time when parties were the reason for formal dance presentations. In France, Charles VI, Louis XIII, Louis XIV, and Henri of Navarre are said to have filled the sixteenth and seventeenth centuries with festivities that made great spectacle of ballet; ballet, that is, fettered with high court costumes and slow, stiff steps.

Ballet was on its way to a separate identity when it moved to the opera. Although still bundled in the fashion of the day, the dances began to become an art, thanks to composers such as Jean Baptiste

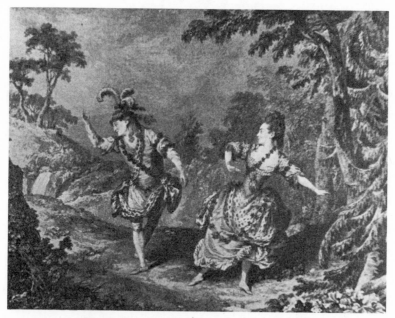

Fɪɢ. 1. Early eighteenth-century ballet costume

Lully and Jean Phillippe Rameau who made some important changes. For one, they included women in the companies. Previously, only men had danced in the mime dances using masks (another confining bit of paraphernalia) to help the audience conjure up female images. For another, they elevated the ballet to a musical level that would be expanded later as dance was taken even more seriously as an art.

It was the eighteenth century before the dancers discarded the high-heel shoes and the long, layered skirts. And it was in that century that the steps we identify with ballet were invented. Until this time the term "ballet" had meant simply a large stage spectacle in which the moving body was of prime importance.

It was Marie Sallé who in 1734 had the nerve to remove her head-dress and bulky pannier and appear before an audience in nothing more than a Greek muslin robe. Throughout the history of art, literature, and dance you will notice a frequent return to the ideas and customs of the early Greeks. Artists associate naturalness, a clean line, and sincerity with that age of man. There are three important dancers in history who looked to ancient Greece for inspiration.

Sallé was the first. Her contemporary, Marie Camargo, invented tights, and the step that crosses the feet several times in the air (the *entrechat à quatre*). We take both of these innovations for granted today, but at that time each was a brave idea. We cannot be too grateful to Camargo for giving us the tights. Anyone who has forgotten these precious items and had to dance barelegged in class knows how tights provide freedom of movement as nothing else can—psychological freedom as well as physical.

Perhaps the most radical reform in ballet came in 1760 when Jean Georges Noverre, the famous ballet master, published a treatise on ballet forms called *Lettres sur la danse et les ballets*. He told the world in this publication that dance should return to the simple, honest forms of nature and not give way to the spectacle of fashion and superficial display of virtuosity. The dance should tell a story with the purest of movement, and the dancers should dress simply so that the body could express itself along its most natural lines.

Noverre's ideas were slow to be adopted and indeed never were in their complete form. Two centuries later Isadora Duncan would be saying the same thing.

Several of Noverre's star pupils added to the current language of ballet, inventing steps we have seen done in every classical performance. Mlle Heinel is associated with the *pirouette*, a step that could never have been executed in the high heels and clothes of the

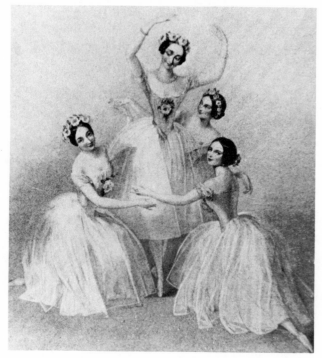

FIG. 2. Marie Taglioni on toe in *Pas de Quatre*, 1845

early ballet. We can thank a man by the name of Pierre Gardel for doing away with the leather masks.

A summary of the changes advocated by these rebels can be seen in a lithograph of Madeleine Guimard. She is dressed in a gently flowing skirt, with her hair hanging loosely down her back. The fact that her biography was written at the time is one indication of the importance her contemporaries placed on her innovations.

While all of this change was going on in France, England was also developing an interest in ballet. In 1702 a drama in dance, the first performance ever without a word spoken, was performed at the Drury Lane Theatre. It was called *The Tavern Bilkens*, and is said to have been the first all-movement show since the time of the Roman emperors. England would later wind up being an important center of ballet.

The grand age of ballet was about to come, and like the great modern dance of this century, ballet of the 1800's was a statement of the thinking and values of the time. We tend to think of nineteenth-century ballet as antithetical to the inner search for honest expression that we espouse in this century, because it is not visceral, and it avoids subjects that reflect the darker side of the human experience. But when ballet is seen against the background within which it developed (and nothing can accurately be judged in any other way), it appears as a vehicle for saying things about life that were of the greatest urgency to the thinkers of the time.

It was a time of Romanticism, a time when life was most validly regarded by looking to the past, through a haze marked with strange wanderings of the mind. An emotional description of life was more highly regarded than an objective one; the simple, unpretentious, individual way of doing things was preferred over the complex ornamented one; the dehumanizing facets of industrial progress were regarded as a great deal less progressive than a return to the rougher ways of living with nature.

At twilight when a thin line of mist settles several feet above the grass and links one side of the woods to another, you can see only the gray blues beyond the mist; your eyes settled there and ponder the translucence. Such a scene delighted the Romantics. Not to see the facts too starkly; to wash the experience in a ghosty, remote simile; to deal not with grand personages and heroic plots but with little people and the importance of their lives; to look beyond the present to a time irretrievable and not quite real—all of this was Romanticism.

All of this was also ballet. And it was the toe shoe that achieved it. On the eve of this profound change in dance, the costume had settled as a dress hemmed just above the ankle and moving out from the waist to allow greater freedom of movement for the limbs. The neck was cut low and the hair was usually wreathed. The sandals that were part of this costume would probably have remained the dancing shoe of ballet if it had not been for the ingenuity of one of the most famous dancers of all time, Marie Taglioni. Pictures of her in 1827 show her balanced delicately on the very tip of her toe, a feat impossible without the use of a special sandal with a reinforced, strengthened tip. Taglioni set a fashion for ballet that has dictated all of the compositions since and that today is at times the one single element that distinguishes ballet from modern dance.

The toe shoe was perfect for the expression of the time. It allowed the dancer to look as if she were not a part of the earth. She was floating off somewhere else in a never-never land where the metal and grime of everyday life were never found. Technically it was a revolution for the dancer. Now she could turn with a grace never before possible. She could be lifted to float through that gray mist and set back down again without losing continuity.

Important, too, was what the toe shoe did for women's roles in ballet. Men could not wear toe shoes. Their arch was different and could not be forced into the mold that the toe shoe requires. Thus the male dancer was subordinated. He became the leaning post, the balancer, the lifter, the one who made the ballerina's dance all the more beautiful but who was rarely as impressive, however remarkable his leaps and turns, as the female. Women had come a long way since the seventeenth-century days of men masked as women.

The ballerina could now appear disembodied, a nice quality for the Romantic age, which enjoyed its allusions to ghosts and spirits. Taglioni's most famous dance is *La Sylphide* in which she is a sylph from some imaginary land of spirit. Another famous dance from that period is *Giselle*, which includes scenes in a graveyard where wraiths roam.

Taglioni died a very old, poor woman in 1884 and with her went the principles on which she had based her dance. The toe shoe had come in for good reasons, and it had been a means of freeing the dancer to a fuller expression of human life. But it was not to remain so.

The emphasis now was on virtuosity. It was not enough to find the most beautiful poses for the human body or to move as if from another world. Now the dancer must enlarge upon the feats made possible by the toe shoe, must take the dance all the way to daring acrobatics. The skirt was gradually cut shorter and shorter until as much as possible of the leg could be seen as it stunned the audience with its high kicks, whizzing turns, and split leaps. The body remained beautiful; indeed, an unpleasing angle or a distorted bend would have sent the audience out the door.

But the emphasis sped further and further away from the simple grace that Taglioni's technique had inspired. As José Limón once said, the technique had "become so rigid, so fossilized, as to lose the freshness, resiliency, and vigor of its original impulse." Even today, when the ballets of the late nineteenth century are performed, the audience is looking for the greatest display of technical ability. They applaud when leaps are done in breathtaking succession rather than when a statement about some part of human experience has been made with perfection. Too many times the choreography is designed around this display of skill, and the meaning of the dance is lost to the acrobat.

We mention this distinction between what Taglioni had in mind

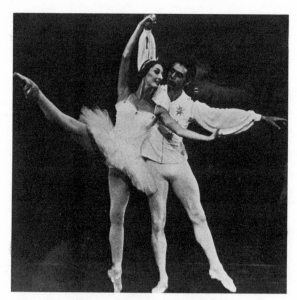

Fɪɢ. 3. Dancer in the short skirt, the *tutu*

and what late–nineteenth-century choreography did with it, not because technical virtuosity does not have value, but because as an educated member of a dance audience, you must know how to experience the performance. When you attend a performance of *Swan Lake* you will know to expect the enjoyment of technical prowess and not to be jarred by the frequent departures from the theme and mood. In the same way, when you attend a performance of *Pillar of Fire*, or other works that stress continuity of meaning in the dance, you will not expect to see sections of acrobatics nor to see an adherence to the classical vocabulary that outlaws distortion and angularity because of their disturbing effect. Knowing what the choreographer intended and from what roots the dance springs are

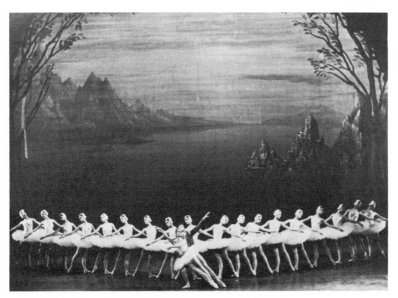

Fɪɢ. 4. Petipa's *Swan Lake*

essential if you are to enjoy yourself fully at a dance performance.

While such choreographers as Petipa, creator of *Swan Lake* and *Sleeping Beauty*, were molding dancers into spectacle makers, one woman was changing the course of artistic history. Isadora Duncan, shoeless, draped in the unbounded garb of the Greeks, hair loose behind her, was letting her body move to the urges within her, to the natural impulses that had for so many years been bound tightly in the tutu and the toe shoe. She was also to hold the rapt interest of audiences in Budapest and Russia and America with nothing to her performance but solo dances danced to grand symphonies. People were awed by her, some were shocked, some were devoted to her, and some were certain she was crazy. But everyone took notice. She had challenged the dance world to stand up for its adherence to rigidity, and for many years she distracted the theatergoing public and got them to listen to her views of aesthetics.

Isadora could not be contained by anything. No rules of the ballet, no conventions of society, no morals or religion could bind her to a behavior she did not believe in. She traveled the world fascinating

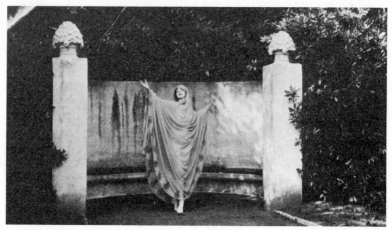

Fig. 5. Isadora in a moment of unchained, upspringing movement

audiences with her unchained, upspringing movement, and she influenced and followed the urges that were inspiring modern writers and painters. She said of her discovery: "I was seeking and finally discovered the central spring of all movement, the crater of motor power, the unity from which all diversities of movement are born, the mirror of vision for the creation of the dance." This central spring was situated in the chest, which she regarded as the place of the two vital rhythms of the body, blood and breath. Isadora felt that "movements should follow the rhythm of the waves: the rhythm that rises, penetrates, holding in itself the impulses and the after-movement, call and response, bound endlessly in one cadence." (*Dance Observer*, Feb., 1934)

She taught young children to dance in hopes that someday dance would flow from a free spirit rather than from the confined rules of technique. And indeed it did, as we shall see in our next chapter on modern dance. We shall look now at the effects Isadora had on ballet; although they were not as extreme, they were important.

One of the great choreographers influenced by Isadora was Michel Fokine. You will surely see some of his ballets that have become standard in various repertoires around the world. They include *Les Sylphides, Petrouchka,* and *Firebird* (*Petrouchka* will be discussed in detail in the chapter "To Die"). Fokine was not interested in abandoning the classical form altogether (indeed, *Les Sylphides* is closer to the classical form than it is to the new moderns), but he did attempt to pull ballet back to the original ideas of Taglioni; to make dance not a spectacle of technical virtuosity, but an expression of the human experience in a fluid, pleasing technique.

Another great dancer/choreographer of the school of thought spurred by Isadora was Vaslav Nijinsky. He was in a particularly good position to cast disdain upon those who danced for showmanship alone because he was one of the technical geniuses of the ballet world. He could outleap and outturn anyone and he was acclaimed the world over for his ability. But his deep personal belief was that dance should go back to its early Greek roots and that movements that most people at the time considered awkward, angular, or flat would be explored for what they could add to the wilting vocabulary of dance. His *Afternoon of a Faun* was a revolutionary piece that reflected his identification with the cubist art that was growing at that time. The dancers move almost as figures on relief sculpture.

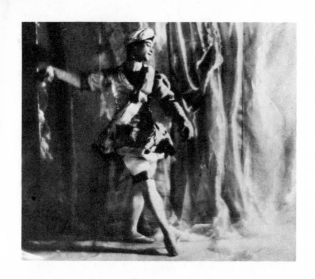

Fig. 6. Vaslav Nijinsky in his *Afternoon of a Faun*

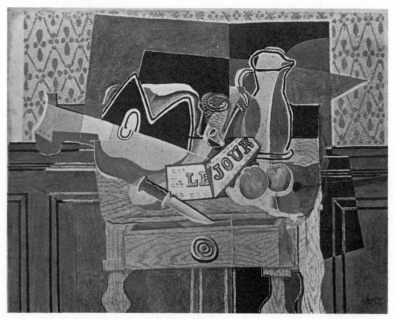

Fig. 7. Cubist painting: *Still Life: Le Jour* by Georges Braque

Nijinsky's life story was written by his wife and should be read for a closer understanding of this great man. One can see in his own drawings, as well as in the pictures of him in his own dances, that his mind was always alive to the designs and tones that the body could express. He was not satisfied to lock the body into a technique within which meaning would eventually lose its identity.

If we owe the birth of modern dance and modern ballet to Isadora, Fokine, and Nijinsky, we also owe it to a man who never danced, but who made dance in the early twentieth century possible. This supporter and indefatigable promoter of the modern ballet was Sergei Diaghilev. He was a rare and important person who could put together complex, expensive productions, charm all of the rich and royal personages into supporting it, and convince the public that what he had to offer was worth their serious attention. He is to be credited for at least three major changes in the world of dance without which nothing we have today would have come about.

One, of course, was his foresight that allowed him to support Fokine, Nijinsky and another great choreographer, Leonide Massine, in their attempts to restore the ballet to its once meaningful place in the arts. The world saw their creations largely because Diaghilev was able to stage them and to move them all over the world. He believed in innovation and was accused in his later career of supporting innovations because they were new rather than because of their quality. But his recognition that ballet would be taken seriously again by the world only if it were allowed to expand, to move out of its complacent rigidity, was a mark of genius.

A second important contribution from Diaghilev was his insistence that music be composed expressly for the ballet. Until his day music for the ballet had been rather trivial and had had the effect of degrading the dance. Diaghilev succeeded in getting such important major composers as Igor Stravinsky, Richard Strauss,

Maurice Ravel, and Claude Debussy to create works just for the dance. Today it is possible to sit through several evenings of ballet in which all dances are set to the music of Stravinsky. Some of the most famous are *The Fire Bird, Rites of Spring, Apollo,* and *Petrouchka.*

Equal in impact with the musical component to the ballet was the development of scenery and lighting. Diaghilev commissioned artists to create sets and scenery that would add dimensions to the production. Such artists as Pablo Picasso and Henri Matisse produced sets for his ballets. The Matisse sets for *The Firebird* are one of the most interesting parts of the work.

In his interest in new choreography, Diaghilev saw the advantage in producing ballets that were compact in their dramatic flavor rather than drawn out through four long acts as was the custom in the nineteenth century. Shorter, more forceful compositions were encouraged, and today an evening of dance will usually consist of several short works rather than one lengthy one.

Diaghilev had his personal problems. Jealousy, ambition, and a passion for novelty, often for novelty's sake, added their troubles to his career. To see him through the eyes of Nijinsky's wife, for instance, who could never grow fond of Diaghilev, is to fill in the spaces in his personality that history so often leaves out. He could be vindictive and cruelly selfish, but his insight into the art of dancing was a contribution we should all realize whenever we indulge in dance today.

Thus, modern ballet was upon us. But today the dances of Fokine, Massine, and Nijinsky seem still classical in flavor and in form. We are used to such moderns as Robert Joffrey, whose dance repertory includes pieces that are as close to modern dance as one can get without taking off the toe shoes. Certainly Joffrey was not satisfied with the changes Nijinsky introduced; Nijinsky didn't think

Fokine had gone far enough in his innovations, and Fokine considered himself a daring revolutionary from the productions of *Swan Lake* and *Giselle* that were shown by the dance companies of his time. The vision to see what else is possible, not to be satisfied with what is currently being done, is the urge that makes the growth of art flourish. So, though we shall always enjoy the beauty of *Swan Lake* and of Folkine's departure from it, we shall also be looking for the newest ballet forms that are emerging from the newest companies.

A lot is to be said about ballet in Europe and Russia, but what about ballet in America? Until 1933 there was no American ballet. We were happy in this country to import our dance, and for a long time we looked upon purely American efforts as inferior, as indeed they were much of the time. But with the coming of Anna Pavlova to America, an interest in ballet was restored, and soon Americans were taking the production of dance very seriously. Pavlova was a tiny, exquisite dancer who charmed her way into everyone's heart as she performed the classical steps with precision and feathery lightness. Nijinsky, too, was beloved by Americans and helped the country plunge into a development of American dance theatre.

The big names in the development of American ballet were Antony Tudor, Agnes deMille, Jerome Robbins, and George Balanchine. The last two are currently directing and choreographing for the New York City Ballet. In 1946 America could claim only The Ballet Society, which was directed by Balanchine. Today there are more than thirty-five professional ballet companies in America.

Of the three companies that include avant-garde ballet choreography in their repertory, the Joffrey is one of the most interesting. Seeing the Joffrey perform is a good way to compare elements of modern dance with those of ballet. A Joffrey performance usually includes traditionally classical pieces as well as new works that

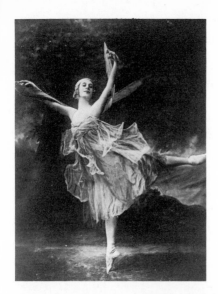

FIG. 8. Anna Pavlova as *The Dragon Fly*

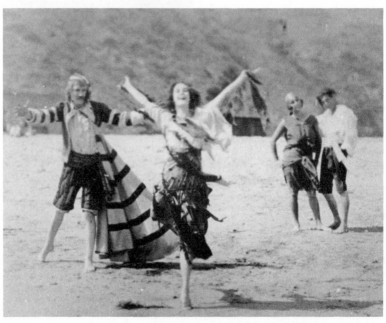

FIG. 9. Anna Pavlova with close friends at the beach

34

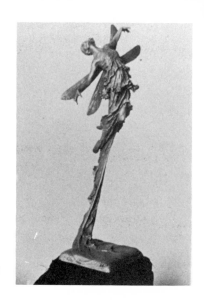

FIG. 10. Sculpture of Anna Pavlova as
The Dragon Fly

hardly seem like ballet at all. But regardless of when or what ballet you see, keep in mind the fact that what you see has grown out of a very difficult and personal history. As you watch the female lead spin freely on her toe, remember the heavy whalebone dresses and the awkward high heels from which she sprang.

Remember, too, that the toe shoes that freed her from that awkwardness eventually came to be regarded as her prison. And while keeping this historical perspective, enjoy every minute of the ballet because it is beautiful and because it fills a need in us to be absorbed in perfection and brilliance and to emerge with a fuller sense of the range of human expression.

35

IV

MODERN DANCE

Modern dance begins with feelings, impressions, reflections, and notions. When the leg moves it does so with enormous conviction. When the body is still it convinces you that the potential for flight is always there. Arms lift or jerk or bounce because they have something to say, not because a formula for movement written down sometime in the nineteenth century says they should move that way. Although there is now a body of skills constituting what is known as modern dance technique, it is never strung together to make a dance. The dance moves out of the mind and feeling-center of the dancer's body and is always a ramification of an idea to be stated.

The dances we shall look at more closely in the next few chapters were built with a fiery adherence to the artistic movement that stressed meaning in dance. These first revolutionaries meant business when they landed onstage with bare feet and contracted pelvises. They had had enough of ballet and its frosty pirouettes, and they were out to change the dance world. As indeed they did. The world was at first shocked, which is a good sign for any new artistic movement. The world was bored at times, too, and felt that its aesthetic sense had been violated. Another good sign. The problem was that modern dance was not pretty. It was disturbing. It seemed to be invading everyone's psychological privacy and to be asserting that dance should do more than just entertain. That was hard to take in the early 1930's.

But fortunately these early champions of modern dance held fast and succeeded in opening the public's taste to dances of lasting consequence. For a moment now we should go back to the beginning to see what was going on in the minds of these artistic radicals, radicals who today seem traditional and solid, though still as lasting in their impact as ever. To begin we must become acquainted again, this time from the perspective of modern dance, with Isadora Duncan.

Isadora

The name Isadora brings to mind a flood of particular images: bare feet; a single body on a giant stage moving to giant music; scarves; upspringing, collapsing, upspringing; tunic; European dancing schools; delicate arms; outspoken candor; soft loose hair. These pieces of Isadora were what the public observed, but what eventually was finalized in those public images were such private moments as butterflies, ocean waves, fiery love affairs, hands on the solar plexus, Terpsichore, resless contemplation, relentless determination, pure vision, junipers.

Isadora is considered the originator of modern dance because she swept down upon the concepts of the nineteenth-century ballet with a certainty that shook the entire dance world. She claimed ballet was stiff, that it did not follow the movement dictates of nature. She in one swoop ravaged the costume, composition, and musical tenets of the day. No toe shoes were to be used, no puffy tutus, no entourage of dancers who form a human set for the premier danseur. Dance was to come from the center of the dancer. Music was to be the grandest. And the costume was to drape over the flow of body lines and accent them. Of the ballet she said:

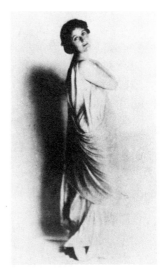

Fig. 11. Isadora Duncan

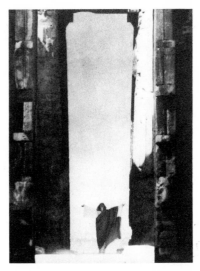

Fig. 13. Isadora among Grecian ruins

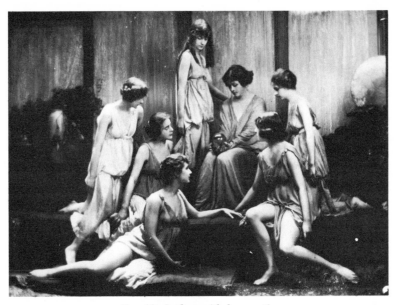

Fig. 12. Isadora with her pupils

The school of ballet today, vainly striving against the natural laws of gravitation, of the natural will of the individual, and working in discord in its form and movement of nature, produces a sterile movement which gives no birth to future movements, but dies as it is made. (*The Real Isadora*, p. 86)

The public reaction to her ranged from adoration to outrage. But the seeing artists of the time saw her for the genius she was and took from her an inspiration and a prodding that would develop into modern dance and ballet as we know it. Michel Fokine, great ballet choreographer of the Russian Diaghilev Company, said of her, in 1905, that he was "mad about her," that the influence of Duncan on him was the foundation of all his creations. Among those creations are *Les Sylphides* and *Petrouchka*. At this point sixty years later after knowing the works of Tudor, Joffrey, Graham, and Cunningham, it is hard to see the Duncan influence in Fokine's dances. But for his time Fokine was a revolutionary, and it is to his work and to Duncan's impact on him that we owe our whole heritage of twentieth-century dance.

Duncan was often accused of having no technique. She claimed this wasn't so, that her technique was different from the ballerina's, but that the place of technique in her work was very important. She believed in gymnastics (a term that in those days was used generally to mean rigorous physical training) and would include barre work as a preparation for artistic expression. She says in her memoirs:

Gymnastics must be the basis of all physical education; it is necessary to give a body plenty of air and light; it is essential to direct its development methodically. It is necessary to draw out all the vital forces of the body towards its fullest development. That is the duty of the professor of gymnastics. After that comes the dance. Into the body, harmoniously developed and carried to its highest degree of energy, enters the spirit of the dance. For the gymnast, the movement and the culture of the body are an end in themselves, but for the dance they are only the means. The body itself must then be forgotten; it is only an instrument, harmonized and well appropriated, and its movements do not express, as in gymnastics, only the movements of the body, but through that body, they express also the sentiments and thoughts of the soul. (*The Real Isadora*, p. 88)

Isadora remains to this day an artist adored by those who seek change, who cherish expression from deepest feelings, and by those who recognize the power of self-belief. Among the things we learned from Isadora is that the conviction with which we act in our lives is often more important than the act itself. To believe in ourselves, to do all that we do with energy and confidence is to hold the power to accomplish whatever we envision. Isadora was rooted in this belief.

Loie Fuller

If the lighting and costume effects of the next dance performance you see are nearly as important to the total effect of the dance as the movement is, you will want to reflect for a moment on a woman named Loie Fuller, who was the first to give serious attention to this facet of dance theatre. Loie created costumes from massive pieces of cloth to extend far into space the natural lines of the body. She used lights to add mystery and dimension to the effects of the costumes and launched the first important statement about dance effects outside the body. It is said that she could make herself appear as an insect. Most of her early dances for which she was in great demand were illustrative rather than emotionally derived. She would dance to depict the delicacy of a butterfly or the flickering of an insect.

She believed that movement should emanate from the center of the dancer, but she was not content to limit the effect to the body alone. The sticks inside the long draperies that covered her arms allowed her to make movements unlike any others being performed anywhere. She could hold an audience for an entire evening. Many tried to copy her techniques, but no one was able to entrance her public the way Loie could.

She was fascinated with the possibilities of light, and worked with technical artists who helped her devise unusual ways of casting shadow, changing color, creating atmospheric movements purely with light and cloth. She kept her secrets well and no one until the work of the Alwin Nikolais Theater of today (fifty years later) has been as successful as she in this exotic use of light.

Her impact on the history of dance was profound. She proved that the greatest effect of dance is not to be found entirely in technique. Its potential is that of total theatre, an idea close to the heart of Martha Graham, who would appear ten years later. She took the audience to lands of movement where ballerinas had never been. And she opened the way for artists who would dot the twentieth century with dances that could not be done without the concepts she produced.

The great poet William Butler Yeats found her dances to be a stirring metaphor for his poem "Nineteen Hundred and Nineteen":

> When Loie Fuller's Chinese dancers enwound
> A shining web, a floating ribbon of cloth,
> It seemed that a dragon of air
> Had fallen among dancers, had whirled them round
> Or hurried them off on its own furious path.

Loie and Isadora were both more at home in Europe than in the United States, since it was abroad that they were most appreciated. In Paris, Germany, and Budapest they received great acclaim as the world of dance in Europe was languishing in those years of the 1890's and early 1900's. Isadora had nothing but praise for Loie's efforts, although later in her life, she expressed disgust at dances that were purely illustrative.

Modern dance can be said to have begun, then, in 1890 when Loie and Isadora, separately and in their individual fashions, set out to clear the stage of bounding ballerinas and to shake the public into an appreciation of the full range of body expression.

Ruth St. Denis and Ted Shawn

The third first-generation pioneer in modern dance was Ruth St. Denis, whose dance has been summarized as exotic and religious, concerned with the spiritual centers in man. And she is, of course, linked always with her male partner and husband, Ted Shawn. We hear often of the Denishawn dancers and the Denishawn school. It was from this first American school for interpretive modern dance that such giants as Martha Graham, Doris Humphrey, and Charles Weidman emerged. Ruth St. Denis was lovable, beautiful to look at, and convinced that every dancer must be trained to dance her own individual dances. She gave strength to the seeds in young performers that would grow toward new statements, new discoveries about movement, new expansions of the range of human expression through dance.

Her dances were inspired by shapes and auras of Egypt, China, and India. Those who remember her remember transparent gold costumes, music from sitars, and bold movement statements about the spirit of man. She had the effect of making young audiences feel

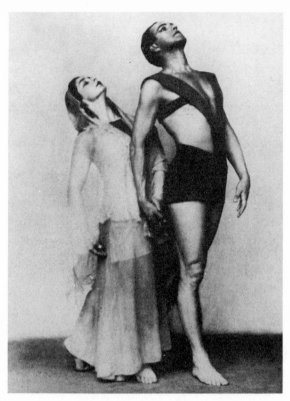

FIG. 14. Ruth St. Denis and Ted Shawn

certain that something very important was going on even if they
had no idea what it was. One of her most famous dances was
Rhadda, which was hailed by critics as revolutionary, exquisite, and
shocking.

Her partner, Ted Shawn, was primarily a dancer and organizer,
and a zealot, not a choreographer. It is to him that we owe the
restructuring of public values toward modern dance as he moved his
company across the country and across the world, exposing the
public to the discoveries that he and Ruth were making. It is also
to him that we owe the progeny who emerged from the Denishawn

44

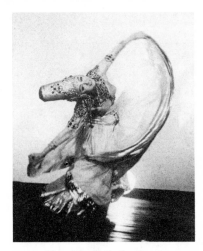

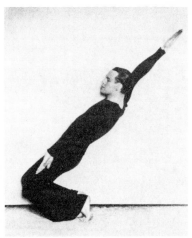

FIG. 15. Ruth St. Denis FIG. 16. Ted Shawn

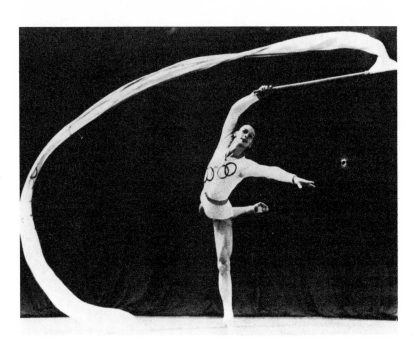

FIG. 17. Ted Shawn

45

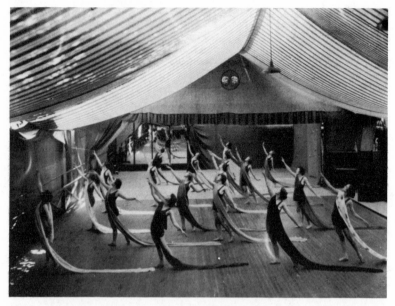

FIG. 18. The Denishawn School

tradition because his energies and foresights created and developed year after year the famous Denishawn school of dance. Schools opened up all over the country and provided atmospheres for individual expression in their pupils that would express itself in some of the greatest dances of our time. Shawn's curricula included as many kinds of dance as could be made available. It is said of him that if there were a Japanese swordsman in town he would be certain that he was found and hired even if for only a short time to teach the art of Japanese sword-dancing.

At times during their careers, Ruth and Ted separated. Sometimes Ruth would leave the company to try things on her own and the group would be known as the Ted Shawn Dancers. And sometimes

Ted left and Ruth held the group alone and in her name. It was during one of these separations that Ted formed his own company of male dancers who were to set a standard of importance for male dancing that had been absent from the dance for centuries. The male was no longer just support for the female. He was finally freed both from that role and from the strictures that the artistic rules placed on his range and variety of movement. The strength, the suppleness, the vigor of the male dancer were finally to be explored. Modern dance as we know it today could not have developed without this liberation of the male.

Still today, at 82, Ted Shawn is one of the forces behind attempts to keep dance a high priority in the minds of educators, writers, artists, and even government. He is largely responsible for the existence of the New York City Public Library for the Performing Arts in Lincoln Center, the only place in the world where one can go to do research in dance and see, without charge, a glorious collection of films of dance. Dances and dancers of the 1920's and 1930's are captured on these films in ways revivals of them will never reproduce. There is even a short film of Isadora, not in her tunic and bare feet, but in a skit in which she at least demonstrates her capacity to be outraged. After a visit to this fabulous film collection one feels a personal sense of gratitude to Ted Shawn.

Charles Weidman, Doris Humphrey, Martha Graham

Out of the exploring, shimmering, exotic world of Denishawn came three of the most important dancers America would ever produce: Martha Graham, Doris Humphrey, and Charles Weidman. Another pair often linked in people's minds, Doris and Charles left the Denishawn company to find their own dance. For both dancers Denishawn was rooted too much in non-American themes. And

47

though the company had given them both the chance to explore movement and choreograph for the company performers (a boon no other dancing company of the time would have offered), Denishawn did not seem willing to experiment with less Far Eastern kinds of dance. They both knew that their contribution lay in other places, and the painful split from Danishawn was inevitable.

For Doris the separation meant the time and freedom to develop her already congealing ideas about dance. But Charles's ideas about dance were still loose and uncertain. At first he was stuck, unable to find his own vocabulary. He threatened to seek the advice of other, more established dancers, but with Doris' frank encouragement returned to his studio to gradually "discover himself."

Out of that room grew dances that delighted, nudged, and penetrated the dance audiences across the country. And, when in 1945 he and Doris broke their partnership, he had attained individual stature quite sufficient to keep him a vital force in the dance world.

When we think of Weidman we think of wonderful hands and a face that danced as surely as did his torso. His finest contributions were comic dances, social commentaries such as *And Dad Was a Fireman, Flickers,* and *Fables of Our Time.* He could also wrap an audience in attention to violence and horror, as in *Lynch Town.* His most singular statement was made in his full-length dance, *Kinetic Pantomime,* which gave stature to the use of purely motor humor.

As a pair, Doris and Charles were perfect complements to each other. Her serious, logical, calculated perception of man was offset by his lighter, more random, scintillating view of us. An evening of dance with their company was a taste of every corner of our experience.

But Doris was to go on to say more, to work out through one magnificent piece after another, her articulation of the natural laws of movement. She had discovered sometime early in her life that by watching her body in the mirror she could discern a built-in recovery system, which meant that all movement is definable in terms of fall and recovery. One need only to stand with head bowed and eyes closed for a few seconds to feel this delicate system at work. Doris enlarged on and exaggerated this law to make her dances. In her own words:

"My entire technique consists of the development of the process of falling away from and returning to equilibrium. It is the exciting danger of the fall and the repose and peace of the recovery." (*The American Ballet*, p. 339)

She is remembered for such masterpieces as *Lament for Ignacio Sanchez Mejías* (which is discussed in more detail later), in which she used spoken words of Federico García Lorca's poem, to create a full theatre experience. Her trilogy, including *With My Red Fires*, *Theater Piece*, and *New Dance*, made up her most complete statement of brotherhood, human passion, and love in an ideal democracy. Her *Dances for Women* and *Passacaglia* will also live as a monument to her creation of new and viable technique and the surge of creative genius that never left her.

A contemporary of Ruth, Ted, Doris, and Charles, but towering above them all, is Martha Graham, the stern, contemplative figure whose dance visions have changed the very course of artistic history. Out of her personal search for how movement makes us feel, she created a new vocabulary of dance that required for its understanding new eyes and a willingness to be disturbed. If we were to hold in our hands for a moment the way in which the human mind works, we would have a three-leveled object. We feel things, we believe things, and we dream things. Martha's dances reflect these

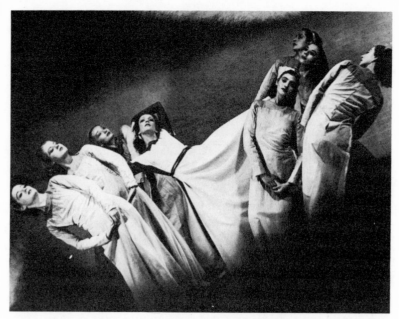

Fɪɢ. 19. Doris Humphrey in *Theater Piece*

three levels of human experience. Some dances seem to emphasize one over the others, and it appears upon reflection of the past forty years that she has moved from an emphasis on feeling things to one on dreaming things. The term dreaming here refers to the mysterious world of the unconscious, which includes the superconscious. It is possible that Martha's interest in the superconscious came from the influence of psychologist Carl Jung.

Three of the dances that emphasized feeling, created in the early 1930's, *Lamentation, Appalachian Spring,* and *Frontier* (all discussed in subsequent chapters) depict moments of intense feeling: *Lamentation* about grief, *Appalachian Spring* about fear and doubt and joy, and *Frontier* about beginning in a strange land. The movements in

Frontier and *Lamentation* are largely pivotal, a product of Martha's sense that dance should be highly contained and organized, never extraneous.

Her dances that emphasize believing include *Primitive Mysteries*, a trilogy based on her perception of New Mexican Christian rites. In three parts, "Hymn to the Virgin," "Crucifixus," and "Hosanna," the dance presents in an almost ritualistic fashion the fundamental construct of Christianity as practiced by the Spanish Catholics in the American Southwest. It is simple and powerfully moving.

Dominating the list of her creations are those dealing with the darker side of the human experience. Images, translucent windings that appear briefly in our dreams, in our mental excursions, and in our fears, are the subjects of a large portion of her dances. Among them is *Deaths and Entrances*, a story of the Brontë sisters that deals with the way memory moves to madness.

Martha's list of dances is long (over 138) and in 1974 she is still producing (although she is no longer dancing, having given up that role reluctantly at age 75). The list begins in 1926 when she made her first public appearance as a choreographer and dancer. But her career as a dancer goes back to her childhood and to her young adulthood when, like so many potential artists, she met with parental disapproval of her desire to be a dancer. Ironically, her father was unknowingly a major influence in her decision to be a dancer. He made a big impression on her when as a child she was caught telling a lie. When Martha asked him how he knew that what she had said was not the truth he answered, "Your body gave you away. Movement never lies." Her parents' objections eventually gave way. In 1916 she enrolled in the Denishawn school.

Martha is said to have been shy and withdrawn at first and Ruth St. Denis told her she would never make a dancer. But Martha's famous sense of her own destiny prevailed, and in a short time she had proven herself capable of the most demanding roles in the Denishawn company.

She was fascinated with the exotic pieces she performed and was intrigued by Ruth's spiritual beliefs. But soon she left the company to find her own way. She, like Doris Humphrey, had a surging mass of ideas to examine and to articulate. Denishawn could not hold them.

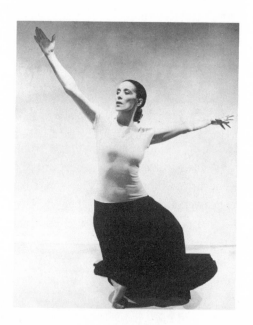

Fig. 20. Martha Graham

Helping her develop her principles of dance, and indeed as much a part of her creations as she herself, was her musical director, choreography adviser, and lover, Louis Horst. Dancers who knew them both have said that Martha's great urge to be equal in her art with Picasso and Stravinsky was kneaded and directed by him. He knew personally all of the finest musicians of the age and kept her ahead of what was developing in the world of music and art.

Following these developments as they occurred, acquainting herself with the most avant-garde thinking, the most advanced way of perceiving the world, kept her dance creations truly in the front of artistic experimentation. Louis kindled her drive and gave it direction.

Martha's attitude toward her work was somber. Her most creative moments were surrounded with long periods of self-doubt, and with the wringing and pounding that accompany the creative process. She regarded herself as a channel through which the force of creativity express itself, and she felt that she could never take time to feel satisfied with her work because there was always something more that could be done. She said to Agnes deMille one day:

There is a vitality, a life-force, an energy, a quickening that is translated through you into action and because there is only one of you in all of time, this expression is unique. And if you block it, it will never exist through any other medium and be lost. The world will not have it. It is not your business to determine how good it is nor how valuable nor how it compares with other expressions. It is your business to keep it yours clearly and directly, to keep the channel open. There is no satisfaction whatever at any time. There is only a queer divine dissatisfaction, a blessed unrest that keeps us marching and makes us more alive than the others.

Merce Cunningham

Since the maturing of these second-generation dance companies (as they have come to be known), succeeding companies and teachers of dance have taken dance somewhat away from the realms of feeling-telling, away from the regions of myth and narrative psychology, and into an emphasis on shape and movement separate from its reflection of emotion. Today in the newer companies we see dances that develop like a modern painting, splashes of line and color, gangling, twisting panels of movement. The first dancer to change the shape of modern dance almost as radically as Graham

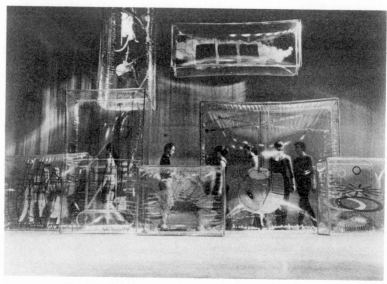

Fig. 21. Merce Cunningham (Cunningham and Co., Wallaround Time [1968])

had changed the shapes of Denishawn was Merce Cunningham. Although his dance creations retain the familiar trappings of stage, costume, musical accompaniment (though never tuneful or melodic), and decor, they defy our conditioning, which has us ready for thematic development, expression of feeling, and tight choreographic construction.

Cunningham's pieces deal with life as it happens, not with life as it feels. You can expect to see movements that you might have made yourself in the lobby before you sat down or in the office that day or in a traffic jam. It is not pantomime; it is a collection of the unflow of our mundane existence. There is continuity and movement, not entirely functional, but it is done in and among movement that reflects what Cunningham thinks of as the happenstance of most of life.

Cunningham started with Martha Graham and danced with her for five years before he left to start his own company and to take dance the giant step further he envisioned. He, like Martha, had his own musical director and one who, like Louis Horst, helped to shape his dances in the light of contemporary musical development. The man was John Cage, and a brief listening session to some of his music will give you a valuable insight into Cunningham's work. No theme is developed, no melody to send you into emotional memories. But there is a linking agent that is primarily rhythm, not toe-tapping rhythm surely, but a relationship between sound and silence that gives continuity to the piece.

Alwin Nikolais

The greatest master of nonnarrative dance is Cunningham's contemporary, Alwin Nikolais. A master of the technical aspects of theatre, Nikolais has turned the stage into a playground of fascinating effects with lights, electronic sound, film, and ruptures of space. He has been accused of dehumanizing the dancer because in some of his best-known works the dancer moves not to express his feelings or motivations but to become a creature of light, of air, or of texture. His dances seem to be insular worlds of their own in which the inhabitants, whatever they may be, carry on the business of living in their own unpredictable bizarre ways. And in that sense the dances are strangely satisfying to the audience.

To watch and enjoy an evening of Nikolais' world you must expect dancers who may represent the energies between light rays, or the flow of impulses from one source of life to another. His most famous piece is *Imago*. Men appear as insectlike creatures and women as bagged sensuosity. It is one of many pieces in which Nikolais distorts the human form by using costuming effect. Arms are elongated, muscles are made to pouch with disfiguring pads, straight body lines are rounded, hard areas are softened. His genius comes through his exploration of the infinite ways the body can appear and move against a sound and visual background that has no limits.

In some ways, a Nikolais concert is an evening of magic, and if you are not emotionally stimulated you are enormously intrigued. In its own way his departure from strictly human themes makes its statement about the sagging, thinning human element in our unsympathetic technocracy.

Alvin Ailey

An evening with Alvin Ailey, on the other hand, is a return to the urges, the joys, the pulsing that is purely human. Originally an all-black company, the Ailey dancers are now the only company in the world that boasts a multinational cast. His dances range in theme; but the majority focus on the plights, the beauties, and the primal experiences of the black man. His music comes from jazz sources, and from the heritage of spiritual songs. The latter accompanies his world-famous *Revelations*, which still brings New York audiences to their feet in wild cheering for more.

Ailey's path has been individual, not a following of Cunningham, nor an extension of Graham. He uses rhythm in his music and

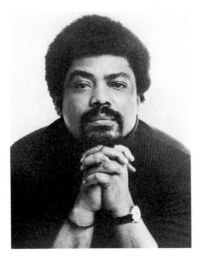
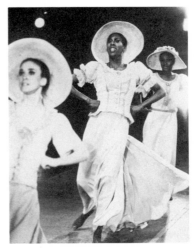

Fɪɢ. 22. Alvin Ailey (Photo: Kenn Duncan)

Fɪɢ. 23. A scene from Ailey's *Revelations* (Photo: Jack Mitchell)

abstraction as well as gesture in his choreography, but the effect is unique, as if somehow melody, rhythm, and movement had never been combined before. His latest work, *Hidden Rites*, dips into musical forms reminiscent of jungle drums and combines silky, patterned wraps of material with nearly primordial movement to send us back as far as Martha Graham ever tried to go in her search for man's earliest motivations.

It has been said that Ailey makes greater use of the space offstage than anyone else, which is really to say that dancers come and go quickly from one side of the stage to the other, giving an effect of windy, energetic, briskly changing patterns. This effect is most radiant in several sections of *Revelations,* and of *Sinner Man,* in particular, in which male dancers rush off and on in one angle and then another, accentuating the fleeing from sin as well as underlining the fast rhythm of the music.

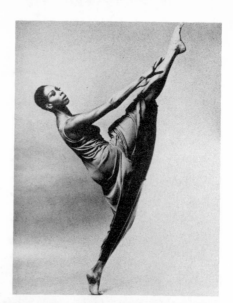

FIG. 24. Judith Jamison (Photo:
Jack Mitchell)

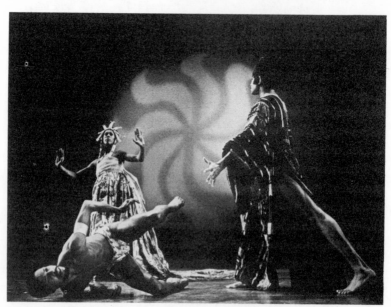

FIG. 25. Judith, Kelvin Rotavdier, and Dudley Williams in Ailey's *Icarus*
(Photo: Jarry Lang)

One cannot speak of Ailey without mentioning Judith Jamison, who is the beautiful, tall, long-legged female star of the company. She is exquisite in the sustained parts of his work and hilarious in the comic parts. She has a way with the audience that has endeared her to all who have spent even one evening watching her. Her tall torso and stately appearance are particularly stunning in *Icarus.* Now internationally famous, the Ailey troupe continues to offer some of the most original work in the dance theatre. Ailey speaks articulately of black problems while wrapping them in a language universal enough to involve every member of his audience.

In the midst of the avant-garde work that takes off from Cunningham and Nikolais is the most hardy link with the past (the past being the ever present Graham and Humphrey genre), the José Limón Company. It was a great loss to the dance community when José died in 1972. Until that time he had been a source of some of the most eloquent, dynamic compositions to be seen in the theatre. His masterpiece, *There Is a Time*, has been filmed with his giving a commentary on the course of its choreography. In the film one can see why he was so loved by his pupils and can recognize the genius that went into everything he did. *There Is a Time* puts to movement the verse from Ecclesiastes ("A Time to Embrace" will be discussed in a later chapter) and captures the singleness of each thought as well as the energy that links each verse to the other.

José was born of Mexican parents and was a tall, handsome figure.

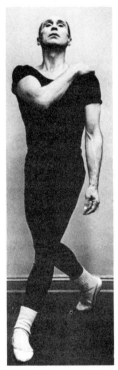

Fig. 26. José Limón

He began his adult life wanting to be a painter but discovered while studying in New York in the 1920's that artists were all struggling to be like Paul Gaugin. He recognized that if he became a painter he would be spending his life either trying to be like Gaugin or trying desperately not to be. He left painting to find a more appropriate channel for his creative energies.

He wandered onto this channel one night when he found himself at a dance concert by Kreutzenberg and Georgi. He was enthralled. He was determined that dance was to be his life, and shortly after he joined the Humphrey-Weidman group in its earliest days. He trained, developed, and became the star of the company for whom many Humphrey dances were choreographed. The relationship between José and Doris was a milestone in choreographic history. Not until that time had anyone broken the tradition of never dancing pieces that had been created by someone else. José, who would later have his own company, saw no problem in dancing Doris' dances, and later the recognition of this attitude allowed dance to expand in ways that it otherwise could not have.

Perhaps the most magnificent role José played for Doris was in *Lament for Ignacio Sanchez Mejías*. In it (the dance is discussed in detail in Chapter IX) he is a bullfighter who represents all enduring, tenacious people everywhere. He faces death with the pride and fight a bullfighter would and then is resurrected by the memory of the woman who loved him. The twisting, balancing, and contorting that mark the dance required the technical prowess of a dancer such as José. His Mexican features lent also a special shade to the piece that another dancer might not have given it.

José's dances, which include *The Moor's Pavane*, *War Lyrics*, and *The Three Women*, are sinewy, and energetic. His link with the second-generation dancers provides a balancing perspective for our modern ventures while his individual style refreshes us.

60

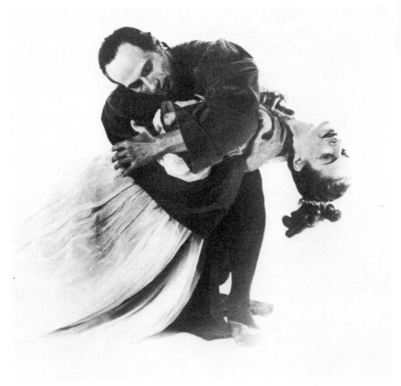

Fig. 27. José Limón and Betty Jones in *The Moor's Pavane*

Modern dance has moved from a nearly violent attack on the emptiness of classical balletic dancing to an experimentation with forms, some of which (as in Cunningham's work, for example) are as far in a different direction from the feeling-center of the human being as the fairyland toe shoes were. The important thing is that the direction is a different one, that dance continues to explore the seemingly endless number of movement patterns the body can make. And the important thing for us to do as appreciators of dance is to

61

experience dance within its own context, to enjoy classical ballet for its attempt at beauty and perfection, and to experience modern dance and modern ballet for the effects they are trying to have whether they be profound emotional involvement or curious fascination.

PART TWO

In the following five chapters we will be looking closely at ten dances, five modern ballets and five modern dance compositions. The dances have been paired according to theme so that the treatment of the theme can be compared as it is performed first through ballet and then through modern dance. In most cases only small parts of the dances are discussed. To explore the entire work would be burdensome and would not necessarily add more to our understanding of the meaning of the dance.

By getting acquainted intimately with parts of these famous works you will enhance your perceptions of dance and add to the pool of feeling you have about the way dance speaks. Your imagination plays an important part in your involvement in the text. Take the sections slowly. Allow time between paragraphs to reflect and dream. The images are there to be savored and to mingle with images that emerge in your mind. Dance works this way, even on paper.

At the end of four of the sections is a discussion of the composition principles of each choreographer. Getting to know the makers of the dances can add new insights to your understanding of their dances. Toward the end, you will see how vast the range of interpretation of an idea is, how limitless the possibilities for choreography.

V

~~~~~~

TO EMBRACE

~~~~~~

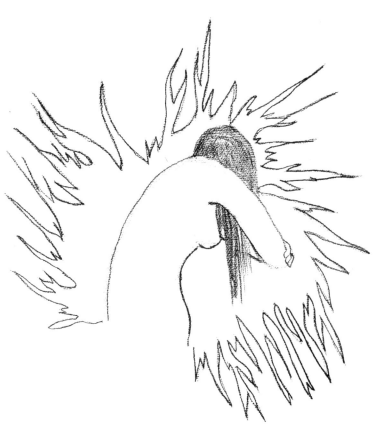

Romeo and Juliet, pas de deux
Choreographed by John Butler

There Is a Time
Choreographed by José Limón

Romeo and Juliet

> Good night, good night!
> Parting is such sweet sorrow,
> That I shall say good night till it be morrow.
>
> W. Shakespeare

That tender moment when two lovers meet, embrace, and express their feelings for each other is a common theme in dances. It is a favorite because it is universal and because it is fluid and easily danceable. When that moment is expressed well, it is a delving into the various feelings that encompass the moment. It is more than joy, more than passion. It is a time also of still appreciation. It has flashes of testing love and of reassurance. It has also the instants of separation that make the union all the more powerful. Butler's dance includes all of these moments, never literally or in pantomime, but through suggestion, through a constant flow that to watch is to remember in our muscles as well as in our hearts what that particular moment is like.

The two lovers in this dance happen to be the most famous lovers in the world. We all grow up knowing Romeo and Juliet. We know that their love was passionate, deep, and tragic. When they met, it was always in secret, and their very coming together was a moment of relief, a time brief and feverish. There was no time for dissension; they didn't talk about things mundane; they had only that short time to bring life to the thousands of fantasies they had had about each other while apart.

Butler's dance is also of two young people as universally you and me as they are specifically Romeo and Juliet. Their feelings are ones we have known.

The gentle anxiety as Romeo enters the room, the joy they find in the very sight of each other, Juliet's teasing, her reach away and quick return to his arms, Romeo's constancy—there are surely no more commonly experienced emotions than these. As the precision of the dancers assures a thing of beauty, so the feelings they are expressing assure understanding from their audience.

Butler's dance has a classical base that only rarely overpowers the feelings he wishes to express. Unlike so many classical ballets, which string together present forms for the sake of movement only, Butler has used the familiar movements as a base from which to deviate in just the appropriate way to make his statement. When, for instance, Juliet with her back to Romeo stands supported by him, we feel comfortable; the position is familiar and the base is secure, but in the next second when she leans backward and to the side beyond the point of recovery, but held securely though gently by his arm, and then looks lovingly into his eyes, we are exhilarated, and the love expression is heightened.

Juliet, like so many of us, had been through years of refinement, learning just how much physical expression was acceptable from a young lady and just where she would be considered gauche and even vulgar. Behind each statement, then, lies a teeming wealth of feeling. It is that quality that is expressed more fully than any other in Butler's dance. As Juliet rises in Romeo's arms, her body facing his, her hand touches his face, and her fingers slowly spread; she creates a delicate moment of withheld passion.

The dance is not just a series of I-love-you's; it reveals also the essential separateness of the two lovers, the moments when Juliet seems to be off on her own somewhere, seeing herself apart from Romeo. There is a motif of this single identity running throughout the dance. It occurs first in a magnificent lift. Juliet's back is to him with her legs straight and apart, from which she turns suddenly into a curled, foetus-like position, nestled safely in his arms. There is contrast between the stretching away from him and the return to her identity with him. The motif occurs again when she falls to the side and is dragged along the stage as if weightless, first on one side and then on the other. There seems at this moment to be no communication between the lovers (less skilled dancers would ruin the effect); Juliet is showing her personality, her virtuosity; and Romeo provides just enough support to make this possible (another admirable trait in a relationship like this); but just as smoothly and as briskly Juliet turns on point and falls into an embrace. They see each other; they have returned to each other as lovers.

A final occurrence of Juliet's single identity is one of the strongest moments in the dance. Romeo is behind her, his hands resting lightly upon her shoulders. The moment they touch, she jerks her shoulders away, lifts on toe to take a second to reflect, then leans again into his arms. It is that feeling of not wanting to say good-bye; of resenting ever so slightly his coming because it must end in his leaving; of wanting not to love and hurt so deeply, to somehow be unsusceptible to such things, and inevitably to acknowledge that this love has transformed her.

The dance works because of the variations of embrace that steal a moment from gravity, that cannot last because they are on the peak of a breath and thereby reflect the transience of the moment. The two most powerful embraces, deriving power from their delicacy, find Romeo on his knees and Juliet resting in four variations on his thighs. At one point she is in an arabesque with the supporting leg resting on his; their necks touch and we feel as if they have embraced. At another point her torso rests on his, her toes touching the step and together they lean closer and closer to the floor. The embrace is moving because our muscles respond to the tentative nature of their balance.

Juliet has her coy moments, too. First, at the beginning when Romeo arrives, she pretends for just a minute to be shy, another understatement of her passion. He must follow her and finally touch her and let their eyes meet. A second time, verging on that piece of cruelty in all lovers, Juliet, nestled again on his thighs, dances with her arms and torso far above him, looking out into a someplace else, a place that is conscious of his suffering, his longing to regain her, and that is convincingly separate from him. Juliet is teasing him, but Romeo is serious. Juliet had that reaction in mind all along. Romeo looks wistfully up at her, his neck tense, adding to the message of his discomfort. Finally she returns to him for another convincing embrace.

The dance ends with a repeat of the luscious side lean into his arm, which restates her love and her dependence on him. As he leaves, she senses the loneliness that is a source both of pain and of joy. She returns to her opening position to meet him, perhaps in dreams, to wait until another hour brings them again together.

In the midst of all the lyrical beauty and the undercurrent of passion in the dance, is the realization always that we don't get to know Romeo very well. He is there at his best when sharing a deep look and embrace with his beloved, at his worst when he seems to serve only as a support for her acrobatics (of which there are delightfully few to take away from the mood of the piece). But we don't see his personality; he is never separate from her; he doesn't tease or taunt her or demand kindness of her. It is this role of the male dancer that so often characterized classical ballet and that modern dance and modern ballet try to avoid.

There Is a Time

It is this role of the male dancer, among other things, that distinguishes Butler's dance of embrace from José Limón's. "A Time to Embrace," a section from Limón's famous work *There Is a Time* focuses upon the male dancer just as precisely and fully as it does upon the female. Limón is never just a support, and when his body does support the body of his partner, he moves into the expression of the moment as colorfully as she does.

Limón's work was inspired by the well-known passage from the *Bible* in Ecclesiastes, 3:1–8:

> To every thing there is a season,
>   and a time to every purpose under
>   the heaven:
> A time to be born, and a time to
>   die; a time to plant, and a time to
>   pluck up that which is planted;
> A time to kill, and a time to heal;
>   a time to break down, and a time to
>   build up;
> A time to weep, and a time to laugh;
>   a time to mourn, and a time to dance;
> A time to cast away stones, and a
>   time to gather stones together; a
>   time to embrace, and a time to refrain
>   from embracing;
> A time to get, and a time to lose;
>   a time to keep, and a time to cast away;
> A time to rend, and a time to sew;
>   a time to keep silence, and a time
>   to speak;
> A time to love, and a time to hate;
>   a time of war, and a time of peace.

The section we shall be dealing with, "A Time to Embrace," has no plot; it is not taken from a familiar story as *Romeo and Juliet* was; but there is no mistaking its meaning. Limón talks in movement about closeness, about embrace in the abstract, but in the most concrete terms. There are feelings in this dance that we saw in Butler's dance; there is coyness, separation and return, looks of adoration from the male, and final parting made necessary by outside forces. But the dances are very different; where Butler's is light, Limón's is rounded and full; where Butler's has moments of "getting set for the movement," Limón's is uninterrupted from the first moment to the last. The most important difference is that Limón in his dance is always a three-dimensional character, as important in the meaning of the dance as is the woman.

A look at a few of the most important movements will clarify this role for the male dancer, which modern dance introduced into the American dance world. When the dance begins, Limón's arms are around the body of the woman in a fashion not seen in ballet. They are there firmly touching as much of her torso as possible. He is not holding her to allow her to leap or fall; his arms envelop her to speak of the essence of embrace. As they sway from side to side, the embrace is deepened and their joy is stated. They move from this simple expression to an elaboration of it. As they turn in place, she depends on him for her balance, but his body moves definitively and with conviction. He is the force behind the movement; our focus is on him. Their eyes look deeply into each other's; they seem to be one person. That mood is not broken as they move smoothly onto the floor. He is still holding her, seeing her, and she moves as he moves. Every muscle is tense, but the effect is one of relaxed interest in each other.

Limón enlarges upon the image of embrace, removing it from the cliché of arms surrounding bodies. Embrace is many kinds of enveloping with many different parts of the body. It is, for instance, a joining of thighs or of chests or of full torsos without ever involving the arms. The moment when she kneels into his lap, when he lifts her by her knees so that their chests rest on each other, and when she rolls onto his torso supporting herself by her own strength, the idea of embrace takes on hues that add to our understanding of it. We kinesthetically recall the visceral component of the feeling that makes two people want to embrace. The extraction and enlargement upon the everyday gestures of embrace reflect more accurately our experience than any number of functional embraces could have done.

There is a moment of adoration in this dance, too; first when he, on his knees and holding her, nestles his face into her torso and she, with eyes on him from above, expresses her enjoyment of his absorption in her. The moment is never still; however, the feeling of stopping time is created by the continuous movement. There is never an evident seam, never a visible preparation for the next embrace.

She, too, must tease her mate, must elicit from him that longing that confirms their devotion to each other. This time it is with steps in a circle around him, holding his hand, moving first near and then away. She explores herself separately from him. He lifts her, holding her at her waist. Her body folds, head and knees touching, then opens, reaching from him, making circles with her torso, enlarging her joy as she touches the air he isn't touching. He holds her, however, and it seems to be this base that gives her her freedom. Like Juliet, she is joyous in herself because she moves through her need for him.

Limón never leaves the motif. When he lowers her they move together always as a unit onto the floor, thighs touching as before, leaning into each other for their last moment together. Others enter to cause their separation; and their reluctance to part is as poignant as that of Romeo and Juliet. It is the woman who ex-

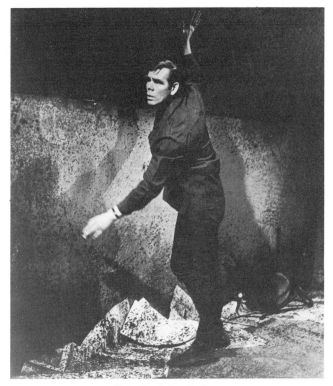

Fig. 28. John Butler

presses the last utterance of sorrow as she gives way to her knowledge that there must also be a time "to refrain from embracing." We are reminded of Juliet's last long look into the space her lover once filled and of her return to a time of waiting.

JOHN BUTLER AS CHOREOGRAPHER

Different from Limón, Butler sees the modern choreographer's role as a widely diversified one. It is not enough, in his opinion, to

73

be just a maker of ballets or of modern dance or of Broadway musical dancing. He must create for all of these and for film, television, opera, and even for society balls. His dance, which we discussed earlier, was created for television's "Bell Telephone Hour" and made brilliant use of camera technique. Butler is not shy of modern media. He uses them for the unique effects each can provide, and his stage is not limited to box-office theatres.

His stage, in fact, can be almost anywhere. In 1955 he produced a modern piece, *Malocchio,* which was performed in the rubble of a fallen building in the Lower East Side of Manhattan. He felt that the setting produced another range of meaning for the dance and heightened the dancers' involvement in the message of the piece. He participated, too, in a kind of moving sculpture at the 22nd Annual festival at Caramoor, Katonah, New York in 1967. Dancers moved in and out of the columned archways, first at dusk and then under the stars.

Butler has choreographed for every imaginable medium. In the 1950's he discussed some of the problems that make each medium a separate kind of challenge. Choreographing for opera, for instance, means that in all cases the dance will be subordinated to the singing and staging. If an interesting idea strikes him for a dance but will require a minor rearrangement of one part of the music, generally he can just forget that interesting idea. Some composers, whose works are new and are perhaps being presented for the first time, recognize that notes do not have to be regarded as immortal and that a choreographer's suggestion for change can often enhance the total effect of the work. But in most cases the choreographer is at the mercy of the musical composition.

Often, too, critics and lovers of opera are unsympathetic with dance innovation that might appear in the opera. While working on the dance for *Die Fledermaus* Butler demonstrated his ability to approach a single problem from two entirely different points of view and in doing so raised the ire of one opera critic. During the waltz, the two principal dancers usually are surrounded by the corps de ballet and perform very classical, floaty types of movement. As a change Butler had the two principals dressed as two parts of a bat and moving as a unit. Then in the waltz scene, he had them suddenly separate to cast a kind of macabre tone over the piece. A review of the opera took special angry note of this innovation.

At a later time he staged the same scene complete with prima ballerina, premier danseur, tutus, and pink tights. Just a different solution in his eyes, not necessarily a better one.

Butler talks also about the problems of choreography for television. Always in this medium, time is the master. There can be no spill-overs, and the dances must be structured to fit into commercial time. This means rejecting ideas that represent elaboration of a dance theme, and it requires, for the sake of continuity, no full-evening compositions. Interrupting *Swan Lake*, for instance, for a momentary plunge into Skippy peanut butter seems somehow more of a jar than breaking into "Gunsmoke" for the same purpose. So dances are carefully chosen for television for their brevity. "The shorter the better" is a piece of advice Butler has often been given by TV producers.

Creating for ballet per se is a different kind of experience. Technically, the problems arise usually from financial pressure. When one is working for the Metropolitan Opera or Covent Garden, money problems are minimal. But a single ballet company, particularly a new one, will face all kinds of interferences because it simply does not have the funds to carry out the ideas that floated pricetagless into the head of the choreographer. Butler has said that the choreographer can choose between dispensing with his idea so as not to compromise, and paying for his idea from his own pocket. Many times he has done the latter. "Many a painting in my collection has left my walls so that I could obtain a backdrop, a curtain, or a set of costumes to fulfill an idea."

Butler, like many choreographers, follows a set approach to creating a new dance. He says that first he settles upon the story line, the general structure of the dance. If the dance has no plot, as in many of his newest works, he settles on the general direction the dance will take. How, in other words, it will get from the first movement to the last and why. He is famous for the endings to his dances and says that they are the hardest of all parts of the dance to create. He can still count ten beginnings that are sitting around in his head waiting for brilliant endings.

Then he chooses the music and the dancers. He prefers to work with composers who create the music especially for the dance so that the two are perfectly integrated. The best arrangement is one in which both he and the composer have the total effect of the ballet in mind and are willing to add or subtract from their respective works to achieve the desired result.

Next he creates the design of movement. He says he does not work out the entire dance before rehearsals as other choreographers do. Fokine and earlier makers of ballet came to rehearsals with the entire dance full-formed in their heads. Butler depends on the music and the artistic peculiarities of his dancers to help shape the specific movements. The result of this approach usually is to have certain roles identified with individual dancers. This is fine, he says, until years later, after the piece has lain dormant for a while and is undergoing revival. The dance will frequently have to be changed to meet the needs and talents of the new dancers.

Finally, Butler adjusts his production to the dimensions of the stage. When on tour he must be aware if stage dimensions will be greatly altered from one stop to another, so that spacing can be changed accordingly. It is ideal, of course, when the problem is an overly-large stage, because sets and curtains can be used to shorten the dimensions. When he moves into a space too small, however, choreographic adjustments can often be major.

Butler, having studied dance for some time, began his career after seeing one of Martha Graham's productions. He was convinced that her work was going to change dance history and he was determined to be a part of that. He looked up her number in the phone book, picked up the phone, and called her. Subsequently he joined her classes and eventually became one of the principal male dancers in her company. His work with her lasted six years. He then moved on, as dancers who are destined also to be choreographers must do, to form his own company and work independently of her style.

Butler's dances have been inspired by such diversified things as a poem by Gian-Carlo Menotti, a mobile by Alexander Calder that moves to indicate the presence of the Holy Ghost, and a woman's gesture that he saw in Italy. He is sensitive to detail that surrounds him and is not afraid to venture into any area in which he finds artistic potential.

His dances can be provocative, though never obscene. Walter Terry has said of him: "John Butler creates some of the most beautiful and imaginative choreographic designs that you are likely to find in the theater of dance. The designs are almost always erotic, and they are always projected by dancing bodies of superb physical beauty. But as erotic as both beings and the movements are, they are never offensive, for compassion, as well as passion, is to be found in Mr. Butler's choreographic explorations of the needs and drives of the human, no matter what the era." (*Saturday Review*, July, 1967)

His dances can also be just as delicate and understated as the one we have seen from *Romeo and Juliet*. As a choreographer he is master juggler of impressions and styles; one who seems to have no prejudices to block his next direction.

José Limón as Choreographer

José Limón viewed himself as "a disciple and follower of Isadora Duncan and of the American impetus as exemplified by Doris Humphrey and Martha Graham, and by their vision of the dance as an art capable of the sublimity of tragedy and the Dionysian ecstasies." His dance moved from the emotional centers of the dancer, and his movements combined to draw a picture, sometimes through narrative, sometimes purely in the abstract, of the dynamics that enliven these centers.

In his teaching he liked to isolate parts of the body and to find as many different ways of moving each part separately from the rest of the body as possible. With the creative insight of an artist, even the head alone can perform a complete dance. Lemón once wrote, "The head can be an erect, proud symbol, or droop abjectly, or roll in drunken ecstasy and abandonment. It is capable of great pendular convolutions, or infinitely contained, minute gestures. Within its orbit it can move in tilted diagonals, tangents, and obliques, which give it a great expressive range." The separation of parts of the body serves both to acquaint the dancer with the kinesthetic possibilities of each part and to awaken new ideas of how to combine isolated movements with larger sweeping ones.

Exaggeration was one ingredient of José's formula of composition. It moves the mundane into the region of art. An embrace, for example, will not look like something you would see in a lover's chamber, but would have some of those lines drawn in movement with larger strokes, with longer phrasing, or perhaps with ten times the force you would see in real life. Another way of exaggerating is to make the movement smaller, to shorten its range, to soften it drastically. This often has a comic effect because it takes the conviction out of it. Wilting arms are usually funny.

Another important element in José's construction of dance was repetition. When the exaggerated movement is done, it is done again and often a third time. Repetition of certain movements gives emphasis to what is being said, allows for an audience who so easily can miss movement phrases, and gives the audience time to see, assess, and react emotionally to it. Movements are sometimes repeated throughout the dance as well as in succession. To recall a movement is to bring that element again into the viewer's mind and to link it to the new phrases; thereby to give it new meaning.

José was fond of bringing the dancer's attention to the same elements of dance composition that appear in the other arts as well. In poetry, for example, repetition of a line or a group of words will have the same effect on the total meaning and impact of the poem as it does on a dance. Two of José's most famous dances (one that he choreographed and one that Doris choreographed for him) are set to poems that make use of repetition for their effect. In José's *War Lyrics*, the lines of a poem by William Archibald are spoken during the dance:

> The women take the blow and bow
> It is done—
> Bow low, bow deep—
> Dig deep
> It is done
> Dig deep—
> Dig deep, dig deep.

And in Doris' *Lament* we hear running throughout the García Lorca poem the line, "At five in the afternoon."

A child brought in a white sheet
At five in the afternoon
A rush basket of slaked lime
At five in the afternoon
A coffin on wheels is his bed
Bones and flutes sound in his ears
The room is iridescent with agony
At five in the afternoon . . .

From the repetition the images increase and the aura of an end, disappearing light, of gradual cooling, collect and reinforce one another to add to the message of death.

José searched for new ways to move that would most adequately express the profound human experience he was concerned with. His movement vocabulary, therefore, never merged with that of Merce Cunningham or Alwin Nikolais. But his range was vast, never limited to prescribed steps and positions the way Balanchine's and even Tudor's are. He was clearly a Humphrey protegé with his own style vibrating from every movement.

VI

TO GRIEVE

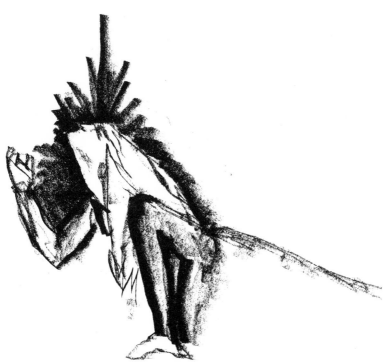

Dark Elegies   *Lamentation*
Antony Tudor   Martha Graham

Dark Elegies

Some emotions can be shared. When we rejoice, when we are amused, when we are embarrassed, we can exchange some of these feelings with another human being. When we do, the experience is often changed; the joy is greater, the embarrassment is lessened, the joke gets funnier and funnier. But when we grieve, we are alone. That others feel our grief does not lessen the pain. It is an emotion, deep and silent, that we alone can live through.

Two exquisite dances touch this reality of grief. They deal with that element in sorrow that is solitude and from which there is no escape. In both, the dancer we shall be discussing expresses the essence of grief; she dances its very core. There is nothing about what caused it; we do not see the scene we usually associate with sorrow, of tears, family solace, attempts to forget, or avoid the hurt.

This is not one particular moment in a flesh-and-blood life. Rather, it is everyone's grief, it is generalized, generic pain. It is a look at lamentation in its raw state; no movement, then, will be recognizable as that occurring in real life. There is no pantomime to draw the study out of the abstract. As an audience we are asked to consider grief as separate from its cause, as bigger than our daily experience, but at the same time as personal and poignant as we can endure.

Dark Elegies, choreographed by Antony Tudor, is a clear statement of grief at its most painful. We are told through the singer's words that the dancers represent the parents of children who have died. The entire community is striken by the tragedy of these deaths, but this cause is immaterial and not essential to the success with which the dance communicates. If you have never been a parent or even have never lost someone very close to you, the depth of suffering expressed in this dance is still clear and moving. In George

Amberg's words: *"Dark Elegies* has a somber, lyrical quality quite apart from the spirit of the subject by which it is inspired." The opening scene depicts in its arrangement of dancers, even before a movement is made, the element that will pervade the work; the dancers, although a group, are solitary.

It is as if they recognize that their mutual suffering cannot ease the pain. This grief will hold firmly and must be experienced. It cannot be ignored or thinned.

It is one of the women's solos that we shall look at closely, as it is in this dance that the solitariness and the confinement of sorrow is best portrayed. Her dance takes place in the presence of the group, each member of it facing away from her, and separated from one another by regular distances. Suddenly she leaves the group, turns with her hands clasped above her face, her head down. She must dance her individual grief.

An arabesque done not as a technical show but as a personal statement reveals the need in her to stretch her sorrow, to fray its ends, to perhaps fill her entire body with it, worsening the sensation, but removing the round pressure from the center where feelings seem to originate and settle. As one arm clutches the other we feel her need to hold on to herself while at the same time her arabesque is telling of letting the body venture away from itself. This contradiction, this needing two opposing releases is a part of lamentation.

A movement that will become almost a motif in this dance is another statement of the undulation from the center of us that we feel when we feel anything deeply. Her arms move in wavelike patterns, first away from and then close to her torso. She brings to mind the sea and the often stated relationship between the sea and us. A Japanese poem that comes to mind during this movement links sadness to the sea in a delicate way:

There is something sacred in salt
It is in our tears
And in the sea.

This movement is done as she moves around the semicircle of other dancers. She passes by each one of them, but they do not notice her. The movement is done also with a step that takes her forward and then backward. Always far enough forward to keep her from standing in one place, but never decisively ahead: another statement of her exploration of the feeling.

She returns to the center, her arms on her chest, her head down. The group has not seen her, and she must live in this moment with no relief. She moves into a reaction almost of anger, but anger mixed with mourning and loneliness. A pattern of violent movements always summarized by a stillness, of looking down with her body in a gentle curve. The frantic turning and flinging of her arms climaxes in a sudden fall to the floor recovered by a lift onto her knees and then into an arabesque, with her head on her folded arms, another quiet summary of her anguish.

She then calls frantically to the world, reaching out into space and moving again from person to person in the group. The momentum of her pacing mounts until the circle rises and she is joined by the others who also mourn. We know even then, however, that the fact that they, too, are grieving does not free her of the inevitability of living through the tearing in her center.

Little in this dance calls to mind classical ballet. We notice the toe shoes, but they are not there to make the dancers light and sylphlike. Neither are they there to increase the virtuosity with which the dancers can perform amazing technical feats. They help to draw an unbroken line from head to floor, to accentuate the simplicity of the costume that keeps the dance as abstract as it is,

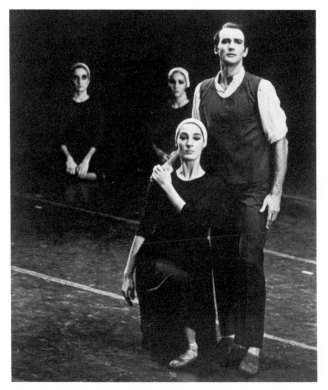

Fig. 29. A scene from *Dark Elegies*—Cynthia Gregory, and Gyle Young (Photo: Arks Smith)

and perhaps to maintain the dance as ballet and not modern dance. We see also a few recognizable classical forms, but their context is intact, and the emotional impact of the dance is never sacrificed for technique. The few times in the piece, when male dancers are seen in duets with the female members, the tendency for the male to be a leaning post and not a feeling member of the dance statement still shows itself, but the moments are infrequent and not strong enough to affect the total impact of the ballet.

An essential part of this effect comes from the music, which does more to accentuate the message of mourning than the words to the songs, which are personal and too intimate. Gustav Mahler's *Kindertotenlieder* is beautifully suited to Tudor's statement about this part of the human experience.

Lamentation

An entirely different expression of grief was created in modern dance form by Martha Graham in her solo work called *Lamentation*. Of this dance Edward Schloss wrote: "Martha Graham does not depict grief, she *is* grief." And if ever an emotion has been given form separate from the human being experiencing it, it surely is in this masterpiece.

The dance expresses human loss as much in its costume as it does in its movement. Martha is cocooned in a fabric that covers her entire body except her face, feet, and sometimes her hands, which stretch to make sculptures of the feelings she dances. The costume is at once the source of grief, the prison in which she struggles, and the bare fiber of the hurt. Hurt is simultaneously the nerves, cells, and muscles that wrench, as well as an energy that transcends these physical responses. As she moves slowly, as if to free herself, she also accepts the casing as part of herself. The desire to remove her senses from the sensors is suggested. But always there is the realization that, ironically, to leave our skin is to destroy our capacity to experience relief. All through the dance the costume is struggled against and absorbed. We see her first plunging her arms into a taut, jersey sea, giving the impression of pushing one's way into a bruise, or seeing inside the pain, which is afloat. Her body sways from side to side in the squat on a single box that completes the solitude we find her in.

A foot rouses itself; it becomes the focus. As it lifts, stretches onto its heel and back again, the hovering body above it seems to be exploring only that much of the sorrow, but she seems to allow the grief to be felt in isolated pieces, as if the pain can be borne when it is not all-consuming. She moves then to pull the cloth tightly and smoothly over her abdomen and up to her chin. She has reached into the pit of her body where grief collects. She doesn't see her center; she has bared it to do what it will.

The isolation of herself in her sorrow is underlined in the isolation of parts of her body from one another. One hand encased in the cloth cannot accept the cries from the other. The bare hand almost caresses the hidden one, but can touch only the cloth that confines it. They do not belong to the same sources. Together they are pain endured in fragments.

Her head, too, seems to belong to space, certainly not to the tiny feet that moved or to the trunk always entombed in the stretched lines of the covering. At one moment her hands move adjacent to her head, which faces toward the ceiling, toward some unhearing relief. The arm moves across the front, her head out of sight behind the arm; the movement is repeated over and over again, the relentless nonpausing that makes up the experience of lamentation.

While isolation of parts of herself add to the desperate attempt to find relief, the unity that pervades the statement and provides the essential contradiction of the experience is seen in her diagonal pull, face looking up, with never a breath taken or a moment of surrender. The grief is there to be seen and felt fully, not to be lessened or coated. These feelings of grief seem to be formed of just these anguished lines and of this narrowed space and of the deep muted color of the fabric.

The dance is perhaps the most fascinating in the history of movement. It is timeless; it is about each of us; it is a use of costume, place, and the body that succeeds in being more than human, in being the stuff, if it exists in time and space, of peeled emotion, while it at no point loses the very real human being who knows the sorrow it expresses.

VII

TO DOUBT

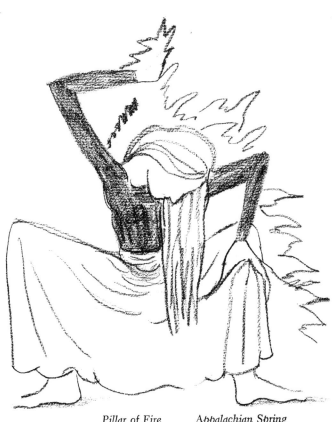

Pillar of Fire
Antony Tudor

Appalachian Spring
Martha Graham

Pillar of Fire

When a young girl grows out of childhood, she faces the realization that falling in love and getting married are two states she must attain if she is to experience womanhood fully. In addition to feeling this, she is aware keenly of the outside pressure on her to demonstrate, by winning her man, that she is desirable. To go through life unmarried is not tragic, she is told, but certainly she wouldn't want to let that happen to her. Even the most professionally minded women consider the experience of marriage. And by the time a girl is 12 a huge percentage of her waking time (and sleeping, too, most likely) will be absorbed in the private consideration of what it means to be loved by a man and to get married.

All young women face this time differently. For many the time is almost programmed for them from the impressions they accumulated from childhood: go to high school, go to college, meet someone a little older, get serious, get pinned, get engaged, graduate, get married. But for some the baby-doll dream eventually yellows. Some must face themselves as they enter spinster age with the consideration that perhaps no man ever will want them. They, in their own fashion, explore the alternatives. When this period of self-doubt is accentuated with jealousy toward prettier, flirtier sisters and with conflicts between Sunday-school teachings and Saturday night parties, the experience can become nightmarish.

Pillar of Fire is a ballet about a woman who must face self-doubt and fear as she comes to terms with her unmarried state. Hagar is about 30, pleasant to look at but not beautiful, shy, and increasingly jealous of her younger sister who seems to have magnetized the entire community of young men. Hagar's older sister is also unmarried and represents the very predicament Hagar wants desperately to avoid. Hagar lives at a time around the turn of the century when rules of social behavior were rigidly enforced by enough of the community to make the rest uncomfortable. These virtuous women move in and out of Hagar's life with their eyes hungry for any morsel of scandal that can be snatched and spread about. Hagar is timid around them and ashamed in front of them, at first of her spinsterhood, and then for her acts of blatant immorality.

Dashing about her also are eligible young men, some of decent reputation, some not. Across the street from Hagar's dwelling is a house of prostitution where men and women come and go, tempting and disgusting Hagar with their pastimes.

Ever present, too, is the man she loves, who, while fascinated by her younger sister's flirtations, is deeply in love with Hagar. She is too uncertain of him, however, to express her love for him and thereby solve her problem. She is paralyzed by the fear that he prefers her sister, that he would respond to her with coldness.

The setting and cast perfectly outline Hagar's state of mind, which is chaotic in its awareness of all the things women can do to declare their womanhood. Hagar expresses her doubt all through the dance until the resolution at the end. She moves often with hands cocked and torso withdrawn, a kind of half-attempt to reach out. She is terrified that she will be rejected, and her bent body and angled arms and hands reveal this. Recurring also is a movement in which she rounds her back, drops her head, and admits the doubt that envelops her. We see this movement as she goes through one difficult encounter after another. A dramatic juxtaposition occurs near the end when, embraced by the man she loves, her head bends as before but this time falls onto his head that has settled against her breast. It is a perfect resolution for her. The movement, demonstrating repeatedly before that she was lost and alone, takes on new meaning as it becomes a means of expressing affection.

A third recurring movement reveals her desperate desire to assert

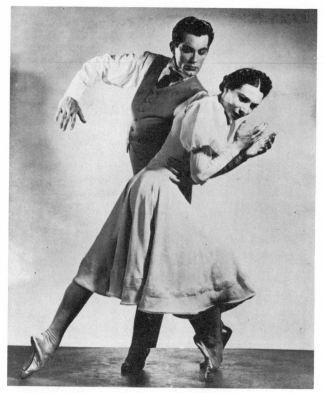

Fig. 30. A scene from *Pillar of Fire*—Hugh Laing and Nora Kaye of The American Ballet Theater

herself and to be noticed by the men around her, but states in the same breath her sense that only within herself lies safety and retreat. She steps forward, then immediately turns from the person in her path, folds her hands on one hip and bows her head toward them.

The most crushing moment for Hagar occurs after she has given herself to one of the men in the house across the street and has run out of the house into the world again. She is flooded with guilt, confusion, and remorse. She falls to her knees three times, bending toward the ground, lifting onto her feet to contain her distress and then runs toward her alarmed sister and falls to the floor. This is the supreme instant of doubting for Hagar. She has given way to her fear of rejection by the man she loves and made love to a man who has no intention of loving her.

This moment moves into moments of disbelief when the man she loves indicates his continued love for her. It is as if she wants to be punished for her indiscretion, to be told finally that she is thoroughly undesirable. He does not feel that way about her, however, and with time Hagar is able to accept his feelings and to move into the forest as his wife.

At that point, Hagar's movements are radically different from those during her period of doubting. They are tall, extended in their lines, and continuous. Her period of doubting is over.

Appalachian Spring

Hagar's doubt as she faced her encroaching womanhood was set amid anxious family, strange acquaintances, prostitutes, and rakes. In *Appalachian Spring*, the set is quite different: loving family, good friends, churchgoers and minister. The dance *Pillar of Fire* took Hagar through a turmoil that could never be a part of the doubting moments of *Appalachian Spring*. We leave Hagar, in fact, where *Appalachian Spring* begins. In this dance Martha Graham is the bride whose moments of uncertainty are couched in the most respectable, most stable environment imaginable. Her doubting is made all the more poignant, because it contrasts with the security that surrounds her. Martha's future is secure; her role as wife, mother, pioneer, model of behavior is assured, and Martha must, in the last moment before she accepts the role, express the basic misgivings that security implies.

The structure from which Martha will flee for a moment is established in the very beginning of the dance with sets of tall, strong lines, sparse but assertive, and with the entrance of characters whose stature is unquestionable: the minister is tall, broad-shouldered, sure of himself; the woman is strong and moves with assurance, almost a symbol of virtue; the churchgoers follow the minister with reverence and conviction. The bridegroom, too, is the very essence of manliness and protective promise.

To understand Martha's few moments of doubting, we have to understand the roots of that security she will examine. Although the time is anywhere and any time, the suggestion is strongly a particular time when culture defined a woman's life in certain terms. Appalachia in the nineteenth century promised hardship in the midst of mountain beauty. Hardship was rewarded by good crops, maybe, and by God's goodwill reliably. It was dangerous to have babies because unattended infection could cause death, but women knew that they would have them and that with luck they would survive to raise them. Days were spent raising, preparing, and eating food, which meant that whatever animals the family raised were tended with as much concern as were the children. A woman contributed her energies to the process of keeping alive and did not question with any seriousness the validity of her duties or her subservience to her man. In return she received his love, his children, and his protection. Alternatives that exist today for young women were not possible then. The food we buy, the entertainment we seek, the clothes we wear, and the houses we live in, all taken for granted in the twentieth century, were acquired in the days of early Appalachia by hand and hard work. Every hour was consumed in the process of getting to the next day. And so a home, a husband, a family, would have represented enviable security.

Martha never seriously considers renouncing these things. But she does remind us of an element in woman's decision to become a wife, which existed just as surely in times of few alternatives as it does today. To marry is to leave your childhood. It is to become the provider of a peaceful home that heretofore had been provided for you. It is to mesh your identity to some extent with your man's, and to bear children whose future will be shaped by this new identity. It is to take a chance on your mutual ability to meet each other's needs and to keep on loving each other while the inevitable change, brought about by growth, or at least by growing old, in your relationship occurs.

Martha's dance is about the doubts that accompany these changes and about the fear with which she looks at them just before she pledges her life to them. The solo (only a small part of the entire composition) occurs appropriately in juxtaposition to the quiet assemblage of bridegroom, minister, and congregation. Their backs are to her; they kneel in the background while Martha breaks away and gives vent for a brief moment to the doubts she is experiencing. She kneels, too, but downstage close to us, and leans over with her hands in prayer as if praying to the land as well as to God.

Suddenly she is up and with little frenetic skips moves about her space, then pauses and turns. She runs back to the group as if to refresh her memory of what lies ahead and dashes away from them again. The skipping reflects the energy, like static, that keeps her moving from one point of view to another. In one moment she looks beyond the present for fantasies of change, and in the next she is drawn magnetically back to the security she senses in the present. She stops, falls on her knees and leans back with her palms raised to the heavens; she lifts to pray again to the land and to God. She turns and flees back to her man, encircles him, and leaves him again.

The stillness of the other dancers with their backs to her and in

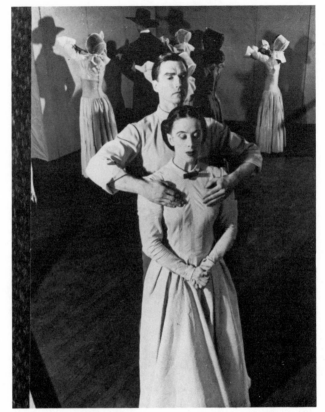

Fig. 31. Martha Graham in *Appalachian Spring*

their silence, increase the separateness of her from them. She must see herself as different from them, as independent for a moment from their society, church, marriages, virtues. This urge rising, she runs again and falls, this time into a split. She twists into a knee-lean and again prays to the land and to God. She races forward; she is farther from them now than she has ever been, and on her face is a look of fear. Her hands touch her mouth. She is remote, alone for this split second with the feeling of being completely separate. Her man rises and moves toward her putting his hands on her shoulders. It is over; she has seen her fantasies for the last time and she moves with her mate to the house and its symbol of domestic strength and protection.

ANTHONY TUDOR AS CHOREOGRAPHER

Recently I overheard the following conversation:

"What do you think of when you hear the name Antony Tudor?"

"I think of a painting by Edward Hopper called *Early Sunday Morning*. Tudor's dances, especially *Lilac Garden* and *Pillar of Fire*, are that painting, somehow. Not that they deal with the same subjects; they don't. But *Early Sunday Morning* makes me feel, makes me react the way Tudor's dances do. It's as if I were there being the characters or the barber shop and at the same time not there,

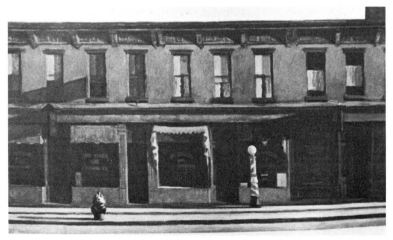

FIG. 32. "Early Sunday Morning" by E. Hopper

objectively reviewing the related images that the scenes bring to mind."

Antony Tudor's best work does seem to have the kind of impact on the viewer that Hopper's painting has. The material seems as real as real life, but its very stylized, slightly defocused elements make it all the more realistic, much more than a photograph could. Early *Sunday Morning is* as distinct from any other time during the week

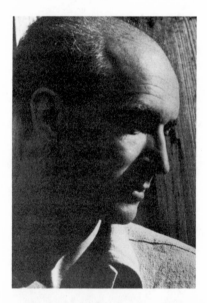

FIG. 33. Antony Tudor

as Hagar's plight is from the divertissements of the other women around her. We recognize both with keen understanding. To study Hopper's painting is to gain indirectly a great deal of insight into Tudor's choreography.

Tudor deals with real situations, real people, real feelings. There is no film surrounding their personalities to keep them safely distant from our own experience. The moment they begin to move it is clear that we will have to accept them into our strange place of painful impressions. It is this genius for creating real characters and for probing their psychological roots that has made Tudor the unquestioned master of modern ballet.

Tudor, taking off in several ways energetically and in some ways ruthlessly from Fokine, contributed a new face to ballet dancing. First, he started each composition with a long and detailed look into the darker regions of his character's mind. The frustrations of deMille's cowgirl, for instance, were dealt with too superficially, for Tudor's psychological odysseys were always slow and serious. Joan Lawson, in her history of ballet, said that Tudor thereby gave "greater depth and intimacy to the ballet."

In addition to the depth with which he examined his characters, Tudor also achieved for them an individuality that surpassed in interest the vague abstractions with which Petipa, Balanchine, and even Fokine works abound. Hagar, for example, is as unique and tangible as Lady Macbeth. We recall her, long after the rest of the ballet has settled into blurs. We remember vivid detail, every facial expression, every change in her torso. She reflects the individual who was anguished, who was subjected to grave fears and doubts about her worth as a human being and her future as a woman.

Tudor's compositions are noted also for their control. Every leap, every brush of the shoulder, every pause is taut and clean. He takes a look from a distance, explores the human emotions in question and turns them into muscular expression and finally into dance. He does not dig from his psyche or his own heart the way Graham and deMille do. He is the analyst, and his work demonstrates amazing depth of understanding. In Tudor's words, "Dancers learned to move in a different way as the visible extension of inner motivation. Gesture was impelled from the deepest sources of the characters, and dance became what an older choreographer meant when he said that there is a region of the heart where words and gestures do not suffice, and Dance, and Dance alone, expresses what cries and actions cannot describe." (*American Ballet,* p. 127)

One critic has observed that Tudor's work contains three separate dance techniques: one is that of the classicist with stylized, controlled gestures, leaps and turns that show roots in Petipa's formulae, and high lifts that require strength from the male dancer and balance from the female. A second technique derives from modern dance with its flexible treatment of body twists, its distortion of classical steps, and its low lifts and low leaps. The third springs from everyday movement. Specifically, from *Pillar of Fire* we remember Hagar nervously smoothing her hair and the women of the town repeatedly picking up the trains of their skirts. Waving, greeting one another with nods and half bends of the torso are also present in his work. The genius he demonstrates is in the synthesis of the three elements. Hee combines them because they are appropriate for expressing the feeling he has in mind.

One dramatic example of this combination within a single movement occurs in *Pillar of Fire* when Hagar in a burst of passion leaps into the arms of the Young Man and is held in a high lift above his head. However, this is no white silky hold he has on her. She is supported with his hand on the inside of her thigh, her hands above her head. "A lift like that would have caused a stampede from the theater in 1890."[1]

Costumes, too, were a new contribution to the ballet theater in Tudor's dances. He dispensed with stiff-netted tutus, swan feathers, and sequined satins. He drew from the street clothes of the day for his costumes and thereby jarred his audience into a more personal identification with the dancers. It was the first time people had seen ballerinas in the very same kinds of dresses and hats and the

---

[1] Rosalyn Krokover, *The New Borzoi Book of Ballets,* p. 235.

men in the very same style of suits that audiences had hanging in their closets.

Throughout ballet criticism, little time is spent in justifying the toe shoe in ballet compositions. But by the time Tudor began his revolution, people were taking a more critical look at the place of the toe shoe in the dance. It is assumed that Giselle and the sylphs must dance on toe for their ethereal effects, and when one settles back to enjoy the pure technician in a ballet, the toe shoe is expected and indeed adds to the spectacle being performed. But when Hagar and her acquaintances danced on toe, some began to try to figure out why. Olga Maynard suggests that "he [Tudor] has used pointe shoes in *Pillar of Fire* apparently to emphasize the feminine nature of the dancer." The very fact that some people began to think about the appropriateness of the toe shoe in ballet was a sign of the profound change Tudor was imposing on the ballet world.

Tudor constructs his dances much the way Graham is said to do. He begins with a situation, taken perhaps from a newspaper account, from a poem, from a legend; he extracts from it the most important emotional and psychological aspects and translates them into movement in his head. He then constructs them and fills in the areas that will serve as supportive background or periphery to the major moments in the dance. Like Graham, he goes into rehearsal knowing that his movement ideas can change according to the particular abilities and talents of particular dancers.

In ballet, Tudor has taken the psychological dance drama to its height. He is to ballet what Graham is to modern dance. To be greater than these two later generations have had to move in different directions, into dance that breaks even their rules of composition, that explore shapes and sounds and disjointed texts the way electronic music and tin-can sculpture have. What has followed Graham and Tudor has its particular kind of exciting validity. But no one can share ground with these two giants in their own brilliantly conceived genres of dance.

Tudor's acquaintance with life at its most real, at its dirtiest, most anguished, most violent surely stems in part from his young adolescence. He was born of poor parents in the slums of London. He went to work as a young boy at 6:00 in the morning to pack meats for the Smithfield Meat Market and worked until 3:00 in the afternoon. He spent the rest of the day playing the piano to earn money for dancing lessons. This combination of activities on a single day, month after month, had related echoes to the work he would do later as the pioneer of a pure art to express prickling, deadening moments in the lives of real people.

Martha Graham as Choreographer

When Martha Graham swept the stage clean of classical ballet form, she replaced it gradually with a form that has since become known as modern dance technique. Her dances, in addition to being tagged as modern dance, have a quality that makes them immediately identifiable as Graham dances. That quality cannot be described in words; one simply realizes after seeing her company and taking classes from her dancers that, in much the same way impersonations of famous actors and politicians are done, one could move in just the right way to be identified unmistakably as Graham-trained. But some things can be said about a few elements that seem to compose Martha's view of dance composition.

First, there are remnants here and there of the classical form. But at just the moment you may recognize an arabesque or a pirouette, she greatly extends it or twists and distorts it in a way that would have sent Petipa into a rage. The arabesque may wind up on the floor with the dancer's head face down; or change into a strange hop that

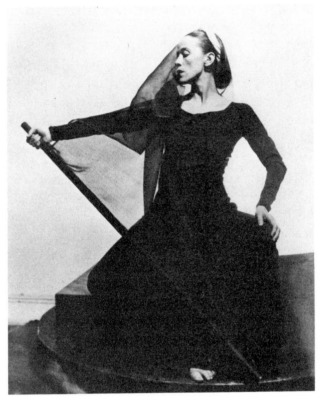

Fɪɢ. 34. Martha Graham

removes any former hint of elegance or symmetry from the step. Here and there, too, are female dancers being lifted by male dancers but never in the classical ballet fashion. Martha's men are not barred by convention from holding onto the female under the arm, on the leg, by the chest or neck or feet. Lifts are not for the sake of beauty and lightness. They are strong statements in which man and woman interact equally to make a pattern in space not possible by each alone.

Her principle of composition is that of the breath sequence. Movement should follow nature in its intake and outlet, in its holding in and letting go of breath. She said in 1934, "The two basic movements are what I call contraction and release. I use the term release to express or signify the movement when the body is in the air and the term contract when the drive has gone down and out; when the breath is out. I do not believe in relaxation. The body should not drop down and become dead."

Martha is adamant about the importance of dance technique in a dancer's preparation. "Every dancer should be concerned with her technique two hours a day as a minimum. If you rely upon mood to carry the dance across, you will soon come to the point where that mood is gone or cannot be recalled at the particular time you need it. If you have no form, after a certain length of time you become inarticulate. The exercises should be done fifty times perfectly, so that you can, when necessary, do them perfectly once. Your training gives you freedom."

Martha at first sought to simplify dancing. She began with a walk and explored it fully. The dances we have discussed are marked by simplicity, by understatement. Often we see just the suggestion of a movement we might otherwise have seen many times on the street. It is cut short; only an outline of it is given. In *Appalachian Spring* there is a moment near the beginning of the dance when the churchgoers rejoice by clapping. But the hands never come together. The gesture is repeated and we know that they are rejoicing, but the gesture is extended in meaning in our minds because it is only a glimpse of the real thing and is therefore fuller.

Martha's dances are constructed with clean lines, never something amiss, never an obstructing image. Even in its greatest complexity her work is meticulous in its form. If a head nods, it does so with conviction and purpose, never accidentally or spontaneously.

To Doubt

Martha sees herself not just as a dance choreographer but as a creator of full-length dramatic presentations. She calls her dances dramas and develops them in light of all of the implication of being a dramatist. Leatherman said of her, "She took over the stage as if nothing had ever happened on it before, and created a new theater and a new kind of poetic drama."

Movement, therefore, is only a part of Martha's movement dramas. She designs as precisely the elements of color, music, setting, and costume as she does the choreography. The general process of her creative work on a dance goes something like this: after an idea for a dance has defined itself in her mind she gives her dancers books, papers, poems, pictures that have led her in some way to this idea, so that they can get a personal feel for what she has in mind. She talks with them about the characters they will become and leaves them periodically to use their own creative intentions, which she will judge later. When she is far enough along, she begins work with her stage designer, another genius and artist/sculptor in his own right, Isamu Noguchi, who will begin design of the symbols/sets to be used in the production. Noguchi has been with Martha since his first design for her in 1935 for *Frontier*. She must also give the script, as it were, to her musical director, who was until recently Louis Horst. Meanwhile, the choreography develops, always changing, maturing, even from performance to performance.

Three or four weeks before curtain time Martha's lighting director and friend, Jean Rosenthal, gets a preliminary peek at the production so that she can begin work on this other crucial element in the drama. Martha at the same time is designing costumes, redesigning them, and making them herself. And somehow, at the same time, she is being consulted on the hundreds of other endless details of production.

The dance builds first out of her conception, from her mental and emotional images, and then from the combination of her dancer's movement ideas and her own. The dance emerges from the feeling within. The body moves always as a reflection of the dynamics between the ideas and the emotion, never as a fancy combination of old, prescribed steps. What she discovers when, as she would say, she "voyages" into herself, she puts directly onto the stage.

She said in 1947 in New York, "I agree with Picasso that a portrait should not be physical or a spiritual likeness, but rather a psychological likeness." Since that time dance has grown into one of the fullest expressions of man's psychological wanderings. We owe the growth of this art to the visions, the solemn moments, and the fiery energy of Martha Graham.

VIII

TO BEGIN

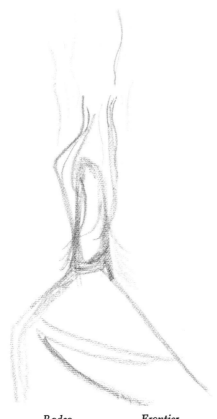

Rodeo
Agnes deMille

Frontier
Martha Graham

Rodeo

For generations the West has been a theme of interest to American artists. And often it has been a theme of beginning. We think of the early days of the West as a place where a family could get a new start in life, where troubled days could be replaced by new adventures, new land, and the prospects for new income. It was a place wide and free where new opportunities were just waiting to be stumbled upon.

The West was also a place where man fought to keep alive under the changeable moods of nature. Without notice, drought could wipe out months of farming labor and leave families with promises of nothing but moving on, to begin again.

But, however grueling the days may have been for those early settlers, come sundown, there was music and dancing amid campfires, bacon and black coffee. Dancing was both a celebration of their steadfast belief that they would endure and a release and time of relaxation after daytime hours of dust and hot sun. Dancers had to be alert to the on-the-spot choreography of the Caller of the Square Dance. Hands clapping, feet stomping in time to fiddle playing, and full-skirted dresses twirling were all well-loved sights that filled the wide night skies.

Even today, square dancing is enjoyed by Westerners. And with every "do-se-do" and "promenade home," memories and sensations of the early days are revived. Although the dancers nowadays leave the dance hall in Pontiacs and Corvettes and return to their centrally air-conditioned brick homes, they do spend a few hours in the evening retasting the beauty of the plains.

Agnes deMille captured all of these Western motifs, all of these attitudes and colors and memories in her first real masterpiece, *Rodeo*. And in drawing on the everyday movements that characterize life in the West, she created a new and highly individual style of

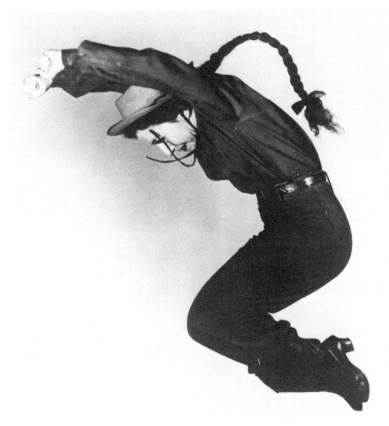

FIG. 35. Agnes deMille in *Rodeo*

dancing. Her characters are real, and through them we become re-acquainted with some of the most charming and ingenuous facets of the West.

The main focus of *Rodeo* is the cowgirl who is dressed like the cowboys, complete with pants, boots, chaps, and loosely fitted shirt. She looks as if she is trying to deny her femininity, to be as much like a man as she can. And her actions, as she challenges the men to roping contests and dances with them to prove her strength and physical prowess, seem only to add more credence to this first impression. But in fact we know all along that she wants very much to be looked upon with love-laden eyes and to be admired for her beauty and her female charms. Her masculine antics are not entirely a cover-up of huge insecurities about getting her man, but they do conceal at first an urgent need to be regarded with as much favor as her rival, the rancher's beautiful daughter.

The entire first scene is spent with the cowgirl impressing the men with her cowboyish feats and trying to figure out how to get their attention in a more girlish fashion. At the end of the scene, the women walk off into the evening and the men leave also in a group. The cowgirl is left with no companion. She is regarded as peculiar by the women and as undesirable by the men. We recognize her loneliness, but her self-assurance keeps us from having pity as we sense that soon she will find a way to fit in with the stereotypes that her society demands of her.

We do not see her again until the third scene (the second is an interlude of square-dancing that adds more Western flavor to the piece), when she is seen still sitting on a bench gloomy and depressed at her predicament. Dancing and laughter accompany the flirting that absorbs the women. The cowgirl is ignored and does not succeed in getting a partner. In a moment she disappears, never missed by the rollicking crowd.

But when she reappears, the situation changes dramatically. All eyes move toward her, and gasps are heard coming from men and women alike. The cowgirl has transformed herself into a feminine creature complete with a blue-and-yellow dress, and hair tied with a large, pretty bow. She moves toward the crowd, embarrassed by their rapt attention to her. Her movements are still reminiscent of a hard-working cowboy, but she tries hard to coat them with her

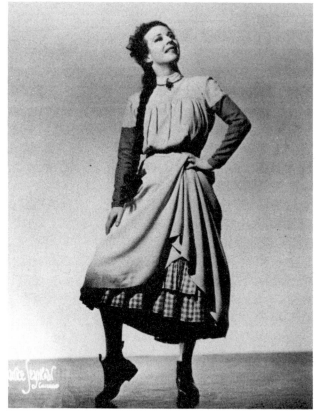

Fig. 36. Agnes deMille in *Rodeo*

feeble sense of feminine delicacy. It is this moment that climaxes the dance and represents her fresh beginning. It is touching, but maintains the lightness that a Western evening of social dancing implies.

She has begun a new role for herself and has succeeded in intriguing the men around her. Naturally she is now with no lack of partners and has the delightful problem of having to choose for

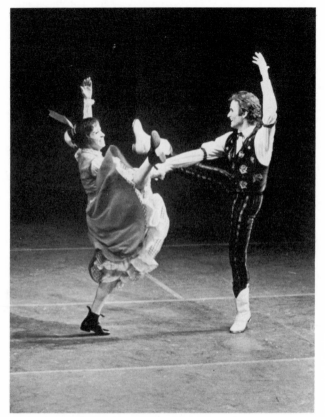

FIG. 37. Terry Orr and Christine Sarry in *Rodeo* American Ballet Theatre

herself. We are delighted when she chooses the roper who has been trying to be her friend all evening.

The nicest element in her transformation, in her new beginning as a female female, is that she does not lose that individuality that made her interesting. Underneath the frills is still the hard-fighting, well-skilled roper and rider we saw earlier. And we sense that fortunately her new man appreciates her for these differences.

To Begin

The dance is permeated with the sounds, the vastness, even the smell of the West. (And the beginning that went on there is, in one of its varied forms, presented with tangible credibility.) While the effect is delightful and gay, the elements of the West are real, never romanticized or exaggerated. It is obvious from the first moment that Agnes deMille was part of the Western life she danced so well.

Frontier

Martha Graham's *Frontier* tells another story of the West, and of a woman's affinity with the land. There are no cowboys in this story, however; no corrals, no boots, very little, in fact, that we usually associate with the frontier. We do see a fragment of a fence, and the vast horizon is emphasized by two white ropes that extend diagonally into space. And there is the frontier woman in her long skirt. But the dance is abstract and depends, as increasingly modern dance would, upon suggestion for its impact. *Frontier* was one of the first dances to leave out so many details and to give room for the wide emotional impact, for deeper interpretation than dances had formerly done. To her first audience, however, this new way of representing a dance about America was somewhat baffling. In Walter Terry's words:

> Of course, in the first seasons the work was performed, there were many who failed to understand *Frontier*. Wasn't dance supposed to be pretty, or, if it had to be serious, shouldn't it tell a story with nice pantomimic gestures everyone could understand? Where was that frontier anyway? There was no backdrop showing mountains and prairies nor was there even a log cabin on the stage. No one plowed and no one reaped and nary an Indian was killed. (*The Dance in America*, p. 84)

113

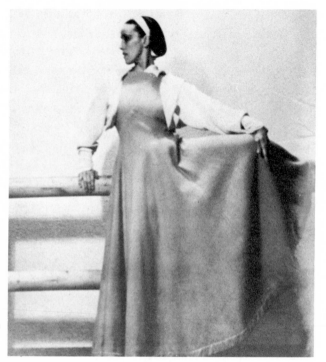

Fig. 38. Martha Graham in *Frontier*

Martha was through with storytelling. She had embarked firmly upon a pursuit of dance that dealt with what was going on inside the characters, not outside. In this dance she *is* the experience of starting something new. She is not a particular woman in a named Western town. She *is* the feeling of having the whole world open up to you, of seeing all potential and of testing its reality.

She is also the bigness, the friendliness, the danger, and the quiet beauty of the West; the kind of beauty Easterners have to get used to—of bare, flat horizons, of lonely tumbleweeds, of road signs that the wind has turned and pointed in the wrong direction, of scuttling horned toads, of white cactus bloom, of empty main streets, of skies so blue you look again, and of next-door neighbors five miles away. Martha dances the feelings that come from becoming friends with the West, and particularly of the early moments when one begins such a venture. When we first see her she is standing with one leg resting on the fence, torso straight and firm as the rails of the fence that support her. She is part of this natural scene, not a human intruder. And for a long time she stays there, turning perhaps to look around but never straying from the position that establishes her union with the land. She seems to be touching all space with her leg and arm as they appear extended farther and farther by the rope that leads into the sky. Suddenly she separates herself from these things and moves with tiny steps into a space less defined. Her tiny steps move as if exploring the range of this space. She makes a square with her movement, a secure, familiar shape. She reminds us of the tendency to create something we understand, to present ourselves with familiar structures when we venture into strange places. And then she moves back to the rail. A test of her reality and a reassurance.

She runs away again, jumping with the enjoyment of her own capacities with the sense that she is part of a vast land, that it will be steadfast for her, that she can look into new ideas, new attitudes, and return with confidence to a land that doesn't change. While she dances away from the rail, the horizon and the rope wait for her, calling out to new discoveries, but never seeking them. She is the discoverer.

"Frontier is a radiant dance of the American pioneer woman, strong, courageous, young and free." Courageous because the land provided the certainty that gives courage expression, free because the clarity of the sky, and the land ambling, slow, and adventurous are hers.

AGNES DEMILLE AS CHOREOGRAPHER

The choreography of Agnes deMille has created a category all its own. It is a new synthesis of classical ballet, modern dance, folk, ethnic dancing, and of realistic gesture. Agnes did something with movement that no one else had done, and the result is a wholly American style. Because dancers perform on toe in most of her work, and because the classical base is always evident, her pieces are classified as ballet. But just as often she is lumped with the musical-comedy crowd because of her famous dances in *Oklahoma, Brigadoon,* and *Carousel*. Actually, she defies stereotyping and should be understood as a separate treasure altogether.

Her style developed as much out of her personal life as it did out of an abstract philosophy of dance which she carried around in her head. As a newly grown woman she was short, stocky, and red-haired (a clear warning to anyone in her way!). That is to say, she was not sylphlike, being neither light nor particularly graceful. She was said to appear self-conscious when on pointe and about to execute a pirouette. And her observation of classical ballet was that it required enormous muscle and strength. She worked desperately hard to acquire these qualities in her dancing, but the result always was more like a swan in galoshes than a lilting feather. America is lucky for this. There were plenty of feathers waiting to be discovered. There was only one Agnes deMille.

She blames her body for her eventual departure from ballet, but her decision was clearly also a result of her strong belief—for many years only a vague intuition—that dances should be "more real, that they should be based on feminine projections with a woman as the central figure," that "symbolism in dance is false to reality."

Soon to surface also was her fascination with Western America, with real problems, real personalities who lived there. The West was in her blood, and many of her finest works drew upon this theme.

DeMille's compositions invariably make use of genuine gesture. Where Martha Graham's dancers imply a clap, deMille's dancers make noise with one. When Petipa's swans hint at a flutter, deMille's cowboys literally get thrown from their imaginary horses. (But at all times she keeps gesture and realism in the context of art; her pieces are tightly constructed, stylized, and purposeful. Olga Maynard says that "of all the American choreographers she has most often and most successfully made use of simple and everyday actions . . . and of genuine scenes."

Her dances require good acting as well as good dancing. The dances must project the feelings that their part requires of them, even to the point of having tears in their eyes. In the *Harvest According*, for instance, the girls stand still, not in the static pose of the ballet premier danseur, but with every muscle feeling the sadness as they say good-bye to their men who are leaving for war. The audience must feel, as we do in a play, that they are real people.

In classical ballet the dance is a "physical or visible extension of the music," and however beautiful, the dancers are not, and indeed are not intended to be, convincing as flesh-and-blood human beings. DeMille's dancers are. In the cowgirl we feel her concrete aggravation at trying to be feminine in a bungling, aggressive body. We can see practically as a tangible entity her need to be loved and the conflicting enthusiasm she has for roping and riding. She loves her horse and her rope. But she also loves her man. And deMille makes us feel her yearnings and frustration.

Not only do her characters move about the stage as real people might, but they also move about on animals as men on animals might. In the first scene the men enter as if on horseback. Their bodies convince us that their feet are not touching the ground and that their horses are spirited. In her first autobiography, *Dance to the Piper* (a completely delightful book that every student of dance should read with pleasure), she describes the difficulty she had teaching her dancers to do this part of the dance. The source of the

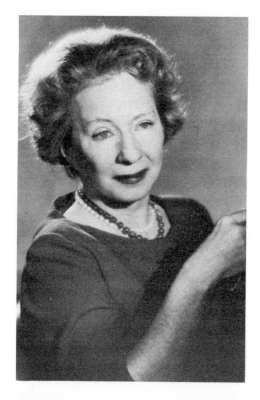

Fig. 39. Agnes deMille

trouble lay in the fact that she was working at that time for the Ballet Russe de Monte Carlo, which employed primarily Russian dancers. And of course the Russians had been trained in the pure classical form. This meant that for years they had worked for hours every day to regard the ground as something you use in order to get up in the air. In *Rodeo* the ground is something you cling to, roll about on, and feel a spiritual affinity with. The ground was more important than the air. Her troupe had no idea what she could possibly be talking about. In her own words, "Up came the delicate wrists and the curled fingers of the eighteenth-century dandy. 'Move from the solar plexus and back,' I shouted, 'not from the armpit. Think of athletes,' I entreated. 'Think of throwing a ball, from your feet, from your back, from your guts.' They had forgotten. They had not used the ground since they were children except to push away from it. Their arms rose up and down but they themselves looked absolutely stationary." She pled with them *not* to plié, but to *sit* on their horse. There is a huge difference.

Ultimately she succeeded brilliantly with the Russians, but not without grave doubts emerging from them as to whether she knew anything at all about dance. In a desperate effort to return to something recognizable and to save this monstrosity from its inevitable failure, one Russian dancer asked, "Might I please, Miss deMille, might I please do some *fouettés* in the hoedown?" She had been told by her Russian masters that she had beautiful skill at this and other classical steps, and she longed to have the chance to show them off. Agnes said no.

Another demonstration of deMille's style as contrasted with classical ballet appears in *The Harvest According*. "For a demonstration of anguish, the women did not delicately bourrée in the agitation of a Swan Queen but fell to their knees, and moved about on their knees, writhing and twisting in an excess of human grief or suffering. The degree of dance technique involved was no less than for the most complex traditional divertissement—only, all the gesture was human, not idealized in classic style." (*American Ballet*, p. 259)

DeMille's treatment of the West has produced unmatched pleasure in her audiences since 1942. New Yorkers, Bostonians, even the

British and Russians respond without need of preparation to the liveliness and the earthiness of her characters. But the fullest enjoyment is experienced by those who know the West as deMille knew it. For them *Rodeo* brings back a rush of disconnected memories of such personal beginnings as sagebrush after a rain, Thursday night dances to *Put Your Little Foot*, solitary hours spent reading a book under a lone tree, a pasture, the smell of sweat on warm, well-worn chaps, and older brothers killing all the snakes in the creek before swimming time. It doesn't take much more than a perfectly executed hoedown to bring back all these images, and in their own way they all have a lot to do with one another.

IX

TO DIE

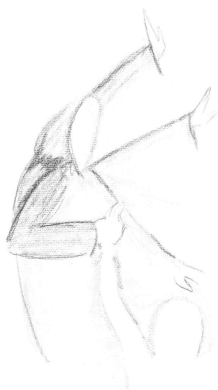

Petrouchka
Michel Fokine

Lament for Ignacio Sanchez Mejías
Doris Humphrey

Lament for Ignacio Sanchez Mejías

If we have not been close to death and survived, or if we have not been through the death of someone close to us, dances about death will be about something else to us. And, usually, they are meant to be. Death is perceived generally as the end, the defeat, the surrender. And though dances about death are about physical dying, they should be seen as a statement also about life.

The character who dies is shaped and has meaning for us because of how he lived. It is his response to death that we care about, not just the fact that in the end he dies. The dance tells us something about his attitude toward himself, about the things that mattered to him in his life, about why he does or does not want his life to end.

The scenes of the two dances we shall look at end in the death of the character. But they are danced as a description of what living meant to him. For Ignacio Sanchez, living was a triumph, a constant test of his ability to stay alive. It was a blur of cheering crowds, and of dust, blood, and lace. For a bullfighter, to die was demeaning. He had risked his life routinely, and to be caught in his own wiles would be supreme humiliation.

Doris Humphrey's work *Lament for Ignacio Sanchez Mejías* gives death a costume and a body, and thereby personifies the force that Ignacio fears and against which he fights furiously until his final dissolution. Without the words or the music the dance is powerful and its message is clear; but the words to García Lorca's poem of the same name as the dance contribute to the total effect the way sets and lighting do. Depth and new images are formed in our response as the words are woven into the choreography. The line, "At five o'clock in the afternoon," recurs and reminds us of the still grayness of that hour, of the impending end of the day, of the dark that is promised, and of the long hours that will separate us from the return of light. That death should be associated with this time of the day is an important dimension in the dance.

Ignacio has been danced (and is filmed) with José Limón as the bullfighter who struggles with the three-dimensional figure of Death and who finally disappears into Death's crevice. In Humphrey's dance, Death holds a coiled rope with which she threatens Ignacio and that symbolizes her link with him. It is at once a means of killing and an instrument for keeping a formal distance between him and her. Death moves about the stage in a long, black skirt, her movements steady, sweeping, and large. Ignacio's movements are frantic and festering, leading in and out of one another as a natural expression of his change of feeling. The set includes a box that suggets a coffin and provides a platform for Death to dominate. Always the pull in the dance is toward this platform at the foot of which sits the long box that will in the end absorb Ignacio.

We see the two figures showing us the power Death is trying to impose upon him as she stands behind him and lets the cord sway above, back and forth across his chest. He is kneeling, leaning backward, his face looking up at her. The next moment he runs from her, but she strikes at him with her rope. His body seems to receive the blows and he waves his arms in defiance. His body curls away from her as his anger builds. A movement that will become a theme in the dance is a kind of striking of the air with his arms crossed, over and over again. His anger must be released, and he is never able to reach her, to tear into her ephemeral flesh as he would like.

Leaping, running from her, he receives another thrust, his resistance for the moment dissolves, and he falls. Each time she strikes at a different part of his body, and his strength slowly diminishes. When he falls a third time she is behind him holding the cord tautly from end to end. That tension bites into the space above his neck, and his head falls limp to the side. Partially crucified, he is on his knees surrounded by his terror that she will not release him.

He frees himself again and runs across the stage to see Death at a distance. His arms cross above his head and then uncross as he taunts her, never leaving her alone, never appeasing her. The conflict within him keeps his struggle alive because to win would be also a surrender.

The dance, then, is a mad conversation with the part of him that fears extinction and the part that steps purposely in the face of it. He unconsciously knows the outcome, but the contest, spun fiercely out of pride and fear, is what counts.

Presiding over the frenetic slashings, over the runs and leaps and contractions that Ignacio performs, is the quiet, waiting coffin and its platform. The structure provides a statement of inevitability that further states Ignacio's conflict.

The dance moves from one encounter to the next in a pattern that leaves us stunned at the end. There are three movements that build the momentum. Ignacio, always in motion, is caught in Death's cord and, almost lassolike, is pulled in toward her, the cord wrapping around his waist. Just as suddenly he frees himself as the cord unwinds. That is the closest she allows herself to be to him and that lasts only as long as it takes the movement to reverse itself and for him to unwind.

Running in circles around the stage, keeping the distance steady, he suddenly falls. The contraction that brings the knees up to the chest is a frequently used movement both because it speaks of inwardness and because it suggests the foetal position, which is a secure, warm condition. That warmth dissipates, however, as Ignacio, alone with his deepest fears, can receive no solace in this position. He must experience that ultimate separation: birth; and then immediately throw himself into the hands of Death.

The most kinesthetically exciting movement occurs after he un-coils onto his stomach and is lying at her feet. He flips onto his knees, and then, with his knees still bent and his arms and head rounded and down, he balances his total body weight on the tops of his rounded toes. It is high, thick, still. The lines converge but never change in Death's smug certainty that he will in the end be hers. He straightens his feet into an arch so that for a split second his entire body weight is on his toes. His agony is beautifully stated here.

He then repeats the theme mentioned earlier of thrashing out at the air with crossed arms, that pitiful attempt to get revenge for the pain and humiliation that the figure of Death has caused him. He moves sideways, embracing his own body, one arm holding his chest and one his pelvis. It is as if his very existence must be held together, and nothing can do that for him; he must gain whatever strength he can by holding on desperately to what is left. Things begin to fall apart as he moves in a syncopated half-walk, one foot dragging be-hind the other, holding on to his fading body.

He begins then the movements that will take him to his death. He edges toward the coffin with his back to it as if a magnetic power were pulling at him, always against his will. He turns in circles and falls onto his knees holding his torso and neck, looking up to the heavens. He is forced by this invisible power onto his feet; and his body moves in fragmented, indecisive, screaming steps toward, then away from, the coffin and the figure of Death, who takes her place near it. Eventually his hands are over his eyes and one arm is stretched away from his body, the hand limp as if in a listless search for relief. Finally his body drops over the coffin, and we see Death in the ultimate dominating position over him. He moves on top of the coffin, never ceasing to resist the power he is drawn to. In the last moments we see a long thin body melting slowly out of sight into the box. A single arm remains in sight until it, too, is gone.

Petrouchka

Although Ignacio has died he will in the next scene return to life to triumph over the physical threats death has caused him to suffer. This treatment of dying is found also in another famous dance, *Petrouchka*, created by Michel Fokine. In this work a puppet comes to life, fights his way half-wittingly through a crippled, piteous love affair, and dies by the sword of his enemy who has stolen his beloved. His death is made all the more cruel by the disregard the crowd has for him when they realize that he was, after all, just a puppet full of straw.

A few minutes later his cruel master comes to drag him away, when suddenly on top of the puppet stand a wild victorious scream is heard and Petrouchka appears, returned from the dead. Immediately he falls again, exhausted, destroyed by his last effort at life.

In basic plot we can see much similarity between Petrouchka's struggle against death, his defeat, his return to life, and that of Ignacio. But beyond plot, the similarities end. Ignacio is a confident, brave, muscular human being whose entire life has been spent proving his manhood. He has fought against the ferocity of the bull. He has turned to crowds and been hailed as hero. No doubt he has been the idol of swooning young women and the envy of young men. When Ignacio dies, he does so with anger, with some fear, and with great energy. In Ignacio we see our determination and tenacity. In Petrouchka we see our frailty. We see the pain that comes with rejection, and we recognize in him profound fear of self. Petrouchka is not bold, he is not loved. He is lonely and afraid of everything, even of the woman he loved. But we care for him just as intensely as we care for Ignacio and probably with more passion.

126

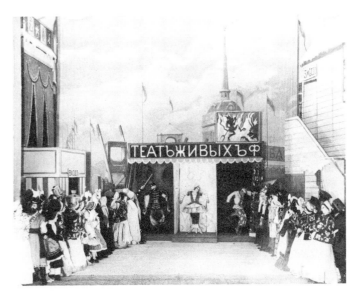

Fig. 40. The puppets begin to move—*Petrouchka*

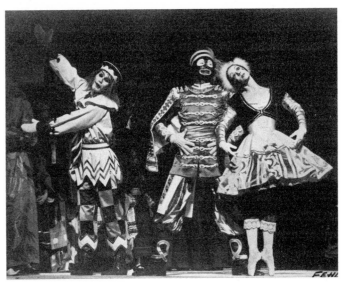

Fig. 41. Petrouchka is sadly different from the other two puppets

In each of us there is Petrouchka's fear that he is too ugly to be loved, that he cares too intensely, that he rejoices too wildly, and that others around him will reject him because he feels with such passion. We love him because he does express his feelings and because his efforts at being taken seriously are always aborted, always

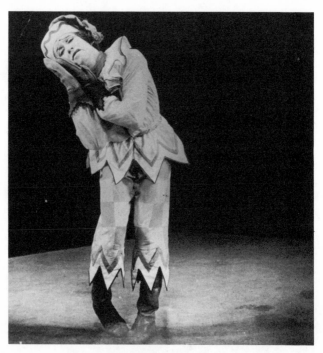

Fig. 42. Petrouchka is alone in his cell

limp and, in the end, just a shape stuffed with straw. Petrouchka's death scene is short but poignant. It is preceded by three scenes in which we have come to feel strongly for him and to take sides with him against his enemy, the ornately adorned Moor; his beloved, the pretty but stupid dancing girl; and against his brutal master, the

Charlatan, who played the flute to give him life. In scene 1 during a carnival, the Charlatan appears, makes plaintive notes on his flute, and begins to move. Immediately we see that Petrouchka is sadly different from the other two. The Moor is dressed elegantly; he is proud and strong-looking but carries about him an air of bestiality, which is a terrific threat to Petrouchka. The pretty, red-cheeked dancer is dressed also with taste and in finished detail. She seems graceful enough, but she is surely not able to produce an intelligent thought. She appears fascinated by the brutish advances of the Moor. Petrouchka, in contrast, is loosely bound; his clothes are not tailored or finished; his smile is on crooked, and his hands are mere patches of cloth sewn together to maintain the stuffing. His body is lank, and his movements are seamless in his frenzy or heavy and slow in his despair.

We know from this first scene that it is Petrouchka's fate we care about. There is a pervasion of gloom around him that prepares us for his eventual death.

In scene 2 we are in Petrouchka's black cell. The only decor is a portrait of his master, the Charlatan, which serves as a bitter reminder that he alone has control over Petrouchka's life. When the door to the cell opens, Petrouchka is thrown inside, as if feelingless, to await the next performance.

The master's foot remains for an exaggerated moment in the door, bodiless, to emphasize the detached nature of his regard for Petrouchka. There Petrouchka moves to show us his disrespect for his shabby body. He disdains his form, which is inadequate to express the glimmer of humanity he possesses. When the dancer suddenly enters, Petrouchka's emotions rise to an uncontrollable peak; he is overjoyed with her momentary attention to him. He adores her perfection and cannot contain his exuberance. But she is frightened and runs away.

We see Petrouchka in a rage, flailing his fist at the picture of the Charlatan who has made him this way. He tries desperately to get out of his cell, but his useless hands cannot turn the knob. His body collapses in a last breath of despair.

When the ballet is performed exactly as Fokine intended it, we are, at the end of scene 2, absorbed in Petrouchka's pitiful state. His movements were choreographed to be loose and inward. His toes and legs, his shoulders and hands were to point toward himself, a means Fokine used to symbolize his introverted nature. The Moor's and dancer's movements, on the other hand, were to be turned out, full of self-assurance. Dancers who are true to this original design produce the stark distinction between the Moor and Petrouchka. Fokine intended, also, that the crowd scenes should be played with great liveliness so that the movements of the puppets would appear less alive. The contrast between puppets and people was to be a major influence on our perception of Petrouchka so that the bite of humanity in him would strike us all the more deeply.

In scene 3 Petrouchka makes his faulting attempt to win the pretty dancer away from the Moor. The scene is in the Moor's cell, which, in contrast to Petrouchka's black one, is decorated with color and elaborate fabric. The Moor shows us his bumbling arrogance as he plays with a coconut the way a baby might, but with a sense that the game is of great importance. He is awkward, and relies for his firm self-image on his unquestionable brawn. The pretty dancer enters and immediately diverts the Moor's attention to her, his new plaything. As he is kissing her, Petrouchka enters, having escaped from his cell by beating down the wall. The Moor is infuriated by his intrusion and strikes out at him. Petrouchka flees. Our affections for Petrouchka increase as we see the haughty Moor gesture coldly with authority to the dancer to rejoin him on the couch.

Petrouchka has become fully human to us. In the final act the crowd appears and busies itself with details of the carnival. Snowflakes begin to fall. The sun begins to set. Into this hectic but rather uneventful scene Petrouchka runs, pursued by the Moor. He cannot run fast enough. The Moor catches him and brutally strikes him

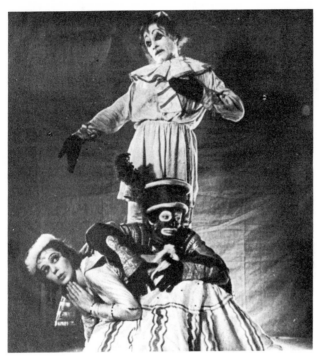

Fig. 43. Petrouchka is enraged and breaks into the Moor's cell

down with his sword. The crowd gathers around Petrouchka's body. We see Petrouchka in his most eloquent movement as he reaches into the air above, seeking some kind of help from a source that exists only in his grasping, struggling mind.

Our attention is turned for a moment to a policeman who rushes

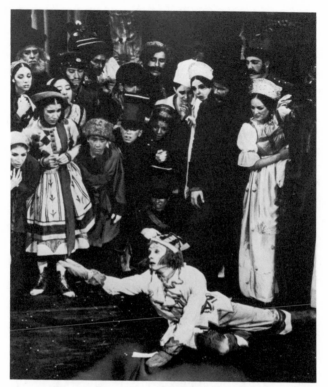

Fig. 44. Petrouchka reaches into the air above

for the Charlatan and to the crowd that stands in horror around Petrouchka, blocking him from our view. The Charlatan appears, to perform the saddest of all movements in the ballet. The crowd moves back, and he leans over to pick up the sawdust doll and show that Petrouchka was only a lifeless puppet. There was no need for all the fuss. But we instinctively know better.

This moment of tragedy is topped by a final one when the Charlatan, dragging the sawdust figure away, is startled by shrieking from atop the stage. Petrouchka has returned from the dead to assert his supremacy over his cruel master. His master flees in terror, but that one last intense effort is all Petrouchka can manage, and he falls, finally, to his end.

We have talked of *Petrouchka* as much in terms of plot as in kinds of movement. But clearly it is not just the sequence of actions that holds the drama of the ballet. In fact, it is possible for *Petrouchka* to be danced so poorly that the impact of the puppet's death is practically nil. Fokine specified movements and attitudes that are crucial to the effect of the dance. And it is notable in this work that very little toe dancing is done. Only two street dancers and the ballerina are on toe, a demonstration of Fokine's belief that dance styles, including toe-shoe dancing, should be done only when directly expressive of the meaning of the dance. *Petrouchka* also includes no virtuoso dancing.

The puppet's delicate link with the human world should always remain delicate. How the dancer moves will make this distinction. In Benois' words, "The great difficulty of Petrouchka's part is to express his pitiful oppression and his hopeless efforts to achieve personal dignity without ceasing to be a puppet." (*Dance Magazine*, 1970)

Choreography matters vitally also in the crowd scenes, which were designed carefully to give the effect of chaos. Bad timing could ruin the effect.

The great Vaslav Nijinsky was the first to dance the role of Petrouchka, and according to Fokine, was the only one truly to understand the part. Nijinsky understood Petrouchka so well, perhaps, because in some ways, he was as misunderstood in his own life as Petrouchka was. He apparently danced the role with a kind of psychological involvement that few since have achieved. "If you look at the photograph of Vaslav Nijinsky as Petrouchka, you see the secret of the puppet's sadness in his eyes. They are wells of con-fusion and unshed tears." (*Dance Magazine,* p. 38)

We can see from discussion of *Lament for Ignacio* and *Petrouchka* two brilliant creations dealing with death. In both it is the character the two parts bring to their death that interests us. In both the choreography has spoken concisely and artistically, giving us some-thing more than a lovely picture to think about.

Michel Fokine as Choreographer

Petrouchka is a perfect expression of Fokine's precepts for ballet composition. Fokine was a revolutionary, influenced somewhat by the revolutionaries of his day. He was very specific about what ballet should be and laid down his ideas in a letter in which he denounced the ballet as Petipa had developed it with *Swan Lake* and *Sleeping Beauty.* He cried out for what he called expressiveness. He wanted movements to mean something, to add to the building of character in the story.

His first tenet stated that ballet should rid itself of "empty flutter-ing," of gesturing and acrobatics. He identified himself with Noverre, who, years before, had said that ballet should not be just "an ar-rangement with grace and precision and facility of steps to a given air," but that it should "study the character and accent of passion and transmute them into the composition."

We hear the same echo, generation after generation, crying for meaning in movement; first Noverre, then Isadora, then Fokine, then St. Denis and Martha Graham. Each was moving away from the one before him, each heading further in the same direction. It is probably true that whatever one is rebelling against in this moment will be rebelled against with just as much fire in the next generation.

Secondly, Fokine called for the elimination of "fixed signs." That dances should be merely a graceful combination of prescribed steps was not enough for him. He looked for the creation of new ways of moving that were based more directly on natural laws of expression.

Third, he wanted to return to the purity of the dance as Taglioni knew it. He saw her not as a demonstrative acrobat, but as one who moved with pure lines to express an idea. He saw her as deemphasizing plot to evoke a mood instead. Fokine sought to subordinate plot, to emphasize, instead, the development of his characters.

Fourth, the components of a dance production should be consistent with one another. Style of movement, costumes, and theme should always grow out of a single source. There should not be insertion of folk dancing if inappropriate. Neither should a dancer go onto her toes unless the added height and weightlessness added directly to the meaning of the dance.

In his memoirs, he wrote, "Toe work I recognize as one of the means of the dance, a more poetic form, removed from the realistic life of some dancing. However, when a dancer jumps and performs feats on her toes unrelated to and unconnected with the subject of the moment, for the sole purpose of demonstrating that she is the possessor of 'steel toes,' I fail to see any poetry in such an exhibition."

In *Petrouchka* we see this tenet in operation immediately. Only two of the street dancers and the ballerina are on toe.

Neither, in *Petrouchka*, is there a demonstration of technical ability for its own sake. This was Fokine's fifth point. No turning or leaping, no balancing treacherously, no splits in the air unless they contributed generically to the dance. "I entirely excluded the turnout of the feet, the dances on pointe and such typical ballet steps as the *pirouette, entrechat, rond de jambes*, as well as various *battements* and the like. *Arabesque, attitudes*, straightening out of polelike legs in fourth position, and the rounded arms over the head—all this was omitted whenever a ballet of mine dealt with

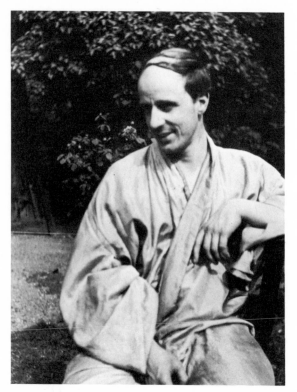

Fɪɢ. 45. Michel Fokine

themes on ancient subjects." The audience should not, in other words, be asked to turn their attention away from the growing impact of the total dance, to be amazed at the technical feats of the premier danseur.

Fokine denounced the choreographer who dwelt on "self-admiration, self-exhibition, and an attempt to please the audience." In his own mind he was the kind of artist who creates a masterpiece because he knows in his own intuitive way that it is right. Certainly it seems to be true that the general public is happiest at first with what is familiar to them. They are not readily pleased with innovation. Fokine knew this, but proceeded without regard for their approval. He received it most of the time, in any case.

Fokine is said to have created each ballet in his head before he taught it to his dancers. Unlike Martha Graham, who used the choreographic ideas from her dancers to contribute to her inspiration, Fokine began rehearsal of his new works by teaching his dancers each step, each attitude, each facial expression as he had visualized it. He worked, also, with the composer and the stage designers and, of course, with the general manager (most often Diaghilev) to complete the work. *Petrouchka* was in fact, such a close collaboration that many critics attribute less credit to Fokine for the masterpiece than they do to Stravinsky, Benois, and Diaghilev. Fokine tells us that when he came to work on the ballet, the story had already been developed by Stravinsky, and the stage ideas already conceived by Benois. It was left to him to create the movement and acting components, which, in the end, are absolutely indispensable.

Doris Humphrey as Choreographer

When we examine the current modes against which Fokine was rebelling, we consider him a far-sighted rebel indeed. When seen in light of modern dance choreographers such as Doris Humphrey, however, he appears slow and all too complacent about the urgent need for an entirely new dance form.

This new dance form we have seen in some detail in our discussion of *Lament for Ignacio*, one of Doris Humphrey's greatest works. In it we see no toe shoes at all (heaven forbid, not even the thought of them!). Movements are not only not a mere combination of

Petipa steps, but also are derived solely from the kinesthetic responses to deep emotion. Her dance is built on her firmly stated ideas about the way dances should be made and has as little resemblance to *Petrouchka* as *Petrouchka* has to *Swan Lake*. Both, however, are powerful and unforgettable. Doris, too, made an explicit statement. If we had had an opportunity to talk with her in person she might have said something like this: "All around you are shapes. Some you can quickly classify into squares, rectangles, circles, and triangles. Some are variations or extensions of them. And some seem to have no category, to be many shapes at once or to slide from one to another. There are shapes within shapes that seem to be at once separate and part of a larger whole. Practice seeing new, bizarre shapes in your minds and transfer them into movement. Within every feeling, every dynamic interchange between human beings, is an implicit design. This design will vary from person to person. Anger may be jagged for you and round and incandescent for me. But shape is always there, and the feelings can be communicated when the patterns they take are discovered. Often, too, we can tell what feelings are being generated between two people even if we are fifty yards away just by seeing what shapes they are making with their bodies. When they form a kind of rectangular box with arms folded and with a distance between them of over two feet, the subject is serious and they most likely are not at ease with each other. Another familiar shape is the triangle that we see when two people embrace and are not feeling safe enough or close enough to let their bodies touch below the neck or chest. Notice, too, the shapes people make in elevators. There are boxes there growing in size with the removal of each person from floor to floor."

Doris would have us first become acutely aware of the shapes around us, as she built her dances partially from this source of design. Although Doris' dances derive from human emotions, they never involve just dancers emoting. Her dances have impact because, like Martha Graham's, they are based on understatement. The dancer who moves in great wailing, in thrashing arms, and in stereotyped chest-beating fails to communicate and leaves the audience cold. There is probably no more poignant, more deeply felt movement in a person's life than the one Doris depicts in *Lament*, but the effect is accomplished by a subtle combination of shapes, dynamics, and movements abstract enough to let the viewer breathe.

Doris was very specific about how dances should be made. They must above all be based on a danceable idea. This means that movement must be a part of whatever is being said. Two men talking over minor family problems at the neighborhood bar is most likely not a danceable idea because no movement is implied there. A man in a fighting struggle against personified Death, on the other hand, is danceable material. The dancer must have a clear notion of the main idea from which the dance will emerge so that every movement will be a consciously contributing part of a whole effect.

The choreographer, when creating more than just pretty steps for pretty dancers to dance, plays the vital role of social-statement–maker. What the dance says about the condition of man, even if it is historically based, will necessarily be a reflection of the choreographer's view of her times. Before she begins, then, she must have come to terms with events, opinions, and artistic statements that constitute her world. Also she must avoid dealing with faddist subjects that can easily become dated and will not make sense to people several years hence.

Important also in Doris' method of making dances was the element of *contrast*. Imagine a house in which all the walls are green; the floors and ceilings are green and all the furniture is green; or a week of nothing to eat but kidney beans, *nothing* but kidney beans; or a library of 7,000 copies of the telephone book. Too much sameness is boring, but it is also dangerous, because after a while the idea that was repeated too often loses the meaning it once had. It takes seeing it in contrast with something else, varying it with differences to keep it vital and individual. You, for instance, are important in this world because you are not someone else repeated. Even twins are individuals, and in their case more than any others', their differences should be emphasized (Hooray for mothers who dress twins differently!). Dances, too, are constructed of contrasts. Heavy movements followed by delicate ones, fast-paced followed by slow, sustained ones. The audience must be given the chance to let one idea take shape, and this can happen most readily if its opposite appears to underline and color it.

Similarly, dances should seek symmetry. Two bodies dancing on one side of a pole with two on the other side doing exactly the same things have too little to say. This is not to say that symmetry is always dull, but it is true that a strong statement intended to make the audience think and react strongly will be most successful in a nonsymmetrical shape. There was a time when scientists believed that nature was basically symmetrical although there has never been a visible sign of it anywhere. Nothing in nature is ever perfectly repeated.

A fourth important theme Doris always kept in mind was the avoidance of flat design. On this subject she said, "In ritual, which has been traditionalized so that feeling is no longer dominant, and in other cold and impersonal subject matter, flat design is the very device to use." She is talking about two-dimensional movement, the attempt, for instance, to look like the figure on a Greek vase or to revive the drawings on an Egyptian pyramid. Dance is to be done with every part of the body involved. If the back is literally invisible, the movement should be such that the audience feels as if they have seen the back.

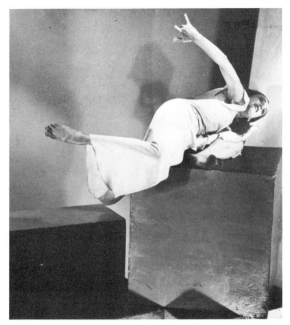

Fig. 46. Doris Humphrey

Finally, movement must be motivated. "A movement without motive is unthinkable." In making this statement, Doris pits herself against history and the present. Petipa ballerinas of the nineteenth century moved with rarely a thought to what they were saying. They were beautiful and that was all. Merce Cunningham and his followers of the contemporary dance theatre are experimenting with a new way of taking meaning out of movement. They make statements about pure movement, intriguing designs, or at times about the "meaninglessness of life nowadays anyway." Doris Humphrey, however, like Fokine and Isadora before her, was tall and adamant that dances should have something powerful and lasting to say.

PART THREE

X

LIZ AND SUSAN

All of the dance choreographers we have considered so far have been from the past. Their works are still very much alive, but those who are still alive are no longer young. It is important, therefore, to complete our look at dance by considering the ideas of dancers who are just beginning their careers, who are dedicating their lives to dance and whose regard for the artists we have discussed will have some effect on the shape of the future. The two interviews that follow are with two young dancers, one a devotee of modern dance and one a ballerina. They are currently facing the realities of the New York struggle to the top and have had some interesting things to say about the people, dance forms, and concepts we have been considering.

Liz Lerman is a beautiful, 26-year-old dancer whose every muscle, every wisp of hair, every thought derives from dance. She believes that dance must come from feelings within, and she is setting out to find a way to create the dances she feels must be created. She expects that her creations will be different from anything we now think of as dance, but they will grow out of the urges and inner conditions of man. Isadora Duncan is her idol—Liz adores her and will exude admiration for Isadora's transcendence of earthly obstacles whenever she hears her name.

Liz has been a teacher for the past three years, one of those rare teachers who elicit from students their very best while never compromising their standards. She left teaching to dance professionally with a company in New York. She wants to see what she can ac-

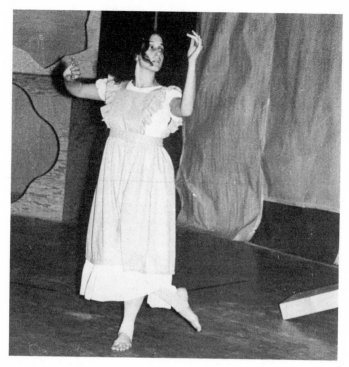

Fig. 47. Liz Lerman

complish when the competition is rugged and the resources for choreography and technique refinement are unlimited. Liz is much more than a technician, and she will not allow those who deny the spiritual element of dance to inhibit her drive to create and dance from her inner stirrings.

*   *   *

Nancy: Liz, you have had enormous success as a teacher here. Why are you leaving and what do you hope to find in New York?

146

Liz: The struggle I have been having with dance for many years is what made me come here originally and is what is making me leave. It has to do with finding a way to move dance closer to its essence, toward that spiritual element that Isadora understood and that has been too often missing in the dances we see today. I have spent too many years going to too many boring concerts where nothing touched me at all. I have taken endless numbers of master classes from the most respected choreographers of the time and found that it was probably good for me because it helped me break out of any movement patterns I had gotten stuck in, but the horrifying thing was that the members of their companies taught us to move exactly like the choreographers did. They had no sense of how not to get in a stylistic rut themselves. I vowed then that I would never get stuck as they had, in my own style or anybody else's.

Nancy: Do you recognize the Graham movement or a Merce Cunningham movement when you see it?

Liz: Oh, absolutely. And the tragic thing is that while teachers of, say, the Graham technique are busily molding dancers to the form and feel of Martha's movements, Martha is (or has been until recently) busy creating new movement patterns out of the real stuff of dance, which is what the dance is saying. To catch a style and hold it still is to destroy the very basis on which it was created: a brand-new way of saying something unique.

Nancy: Perhaps, then, that is why Martha is so miserable when her dances are being revived. The technique of past dances is no longer part of the present and therefore can never be what it was when it was first conceived. It is like asking an adult to become a child again.

Liz: Yes, I think so, and what I want to do is go from here to something still newer, not to merely offer my body as a tool for saying something that has been said over and over. And I expect that I will never be content with being someone else's tool; I will have to make my own dances.

Nancy: But when you first get to New York you won't be able to do that will you? How will it be not to choreograph for a year or more?

Liz: It will be all right, I guess, for a while. But eventually I want to see if the kind of work I have done at Sandy Spring can be enlarged, perfected, and understood by the New York world. I guess first I have to find out if that monster is really there.

Nancy: What monster?

Liz: The loyalty games that keep us from looking for what is central to the individual dancer. At Bennington I was nauseated by the machine-like way they dealt with students of dance; in master classes it was the same way, and I hear that in New York it is like a factory. I want to find out if that is true. I realize that at Bennington I was as closed-minded as they were, and I don't know if the impressions I have of the direction dance is going in are true or are just my distorted feelings.

Nancy: Can you capsulize what you think dance has meant to you as a person as well as a teacher and professional dancer?

Liz: Dance is privately the one way I can be most myself, and publicly it is a way of sharing that. The part of me I have been most aware of for twelve years is my own incredible need to dance. Dancing is the best way I know to integrate all of my life. When I am driving down a road and I see a sign, it transfers itself into a dance.

Nancy: Do you listen to music in the same way?

Liz: No, not all the time. Classical music, like Mozart, I don't because I can't imagine doing a dance to that.

Nancy: How, then, do you respond to classical ballet that is choreographed to classical music?

Liz: I would never choreograph it, and I don't really enjoy an evening of classical ballet, but I do enjoy it from a historical point of view. It is like the way I enjoy a perfectly cut diamond. For its perfection and its beauty I can appreciate it, but it doesn't mean a great deal to me outside of that.

Nancy: Do you think ballerinas and modern dancers are interchangeable technique-wise?

Liz: No, in fact, I had an interesting experience once in London where I saw a dance concert in which two dances were performed by [Rudolf] Nureyev. One was a modern piece by Glen Tetty, which Nureyev could not dance at all. He was terrible. He had no sense of what was going on in the dance. But in the older piece, which he had brought from Russia, he was exquisite. He was perfect. That is the kind of dance he should do because his body doesn't have the vocabulary or the understanding of modern movement.

Nancy: So, what do you feel are the important differences between dancers of ballet and modern dance?

Liz: A fine ballerina is limited because of her training. She may be brilliant, but she is limited. A modern dancer, theoretically, is not limited, and more and more modern choreographers are insisting that their dancers have a good classical background as well as training in modern dance technique.

Nancy: You said earlier, though, that many modern dance companies are also limited, are stuck.

Liz: That is why I say theoretically. There are companies that are not stuck. When feeling and technique are balanced in a choreographer's priorities, exciting things happen. Most often feeling is not a part of classical ballet. Technique, virtuosity dominates. But it is certainly true that technique can dominate modern dance composition, too. Merce Cunningham, for instance, is Graham technique without the feeling. He worked with Graham for a while and then left her. He removed from her the emotional quality. So, when you do a contraction with Graham, it is intense and you have to feel it from the gut. Cunningham, on the other hand, says "round your back." What you remove when you don't contract from the gut is that crucial punch.

Nancy: So, you can't see value in Cunningham's work?

Liz: Quite the contrary. And this is another contradiction in my philosophy. When I first encountered Cunningham technique it seemed arbitrary. (I came from a straight Graham tradition.) I couldn't stand it. I have since come to love it. I have discovered that there is validity in movement for movement's sake. But the other side of me objects to dance that doesn't say something and that doesn't emerge from the depths of the dancer.

Nancy: Will you study with him, then?

Liz: Viola Farber is a split-off from him. I may study there.

Nancy: What was your childhood experience in dance and who were your greatest teachers?

Liz: When I was very small, I was going to be a great ballerina. But I had an unusual teacher, a great woman, Florence West. I remember her teaching us that movement must express something, and she would have us do the most amazing things as part of our dance class. One time she had us make pictures with string and block-print it and then put tissue paper that we had cut up in layers on the print. Then we would work dances on it, creating dances to express something of that picture.

Florence West was amazing. If any person has been responsible for my success as a dancer it has been that incredible woman. I remember her saying that modern dance would have come in much sooner than it did except that they found the toe shoe first and to maintain balance a dancer on toe must keep her torso quiet.

There was another person who had a great influence on me who was not a dance teacher but who knew me very well. He said to me, "If you were a dancer, you would be a cardboard figure. But you're not. You are a *person* who loves dance."

Nancy: As you leave teaching, Liz, what do you feel are the difficulties educators and students of dance face?

Liz: Always it will be the decision of whether to encourage professionalism in their dancers. The problem comes when the dance department of a school deprives the students of the personal interest in what dance can contribute to them as people and emphasizes the standards and detachment of professional dance instead. If they are going to get that they might as well be in New York. And the school has to face the fact that they are not in New York and that their students are therefore not getting either experience of dance fully.

Nancy: Is there one thing you would like to say in your dance?

Liz: I would like to prove with my life that to be an artist you don't have to be neurotic. I don't believe what so many people say about the pathological nature of genius. I would also like to create a new kind of dance, one that takes into account the exciting relationship between sound, shape, film, speech, and movement. Merging the media toward one comprehensible whole fascinates me. I believe that great dance must move in that direction.

* * *

Susan Jones is a member of the American Ballet Theatre whose bright eyes and ability to project to an audience add extra excitement to her ballet dancing. She knows that dance derives from the feelings found in real life, and she puts into her dancing a conviction and authenticity not found in every dancer. Her work with Antony Tudor has added immeasurably to her own belief that the dancer must understand the emotions she is portraying and must work until she has combined technical skill with a true sense of the character she must become onstage. The dancer must be an artist, not just a technician.

* * *

Nancy: Susan, how did you first become interested in ballet?
Susan: Through music, I guess. As a little girl, I always moved to music. My mother used to tell me that I had a kind of natural rhythm that most other little children didn't have. And when I was 5, I started the usual set of dancing lessons: tap, Hawaiian and all of the commercial kinds of dance little children are exposed to. When I was 12, I studied with a branch of the Mary Day's Washington School of Ballet in Rockville, Maryland. My teacher was Lucille Hood. Then I went to the Washington School for

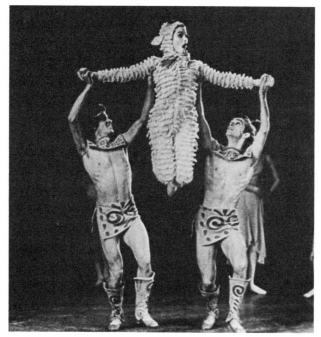

Fig. 48. Susan Jones of American Ballet Theatre

the Ballet in the District for my 10th and 11th grades. When I was 16, I came to New York.

Nancy: Were you able to join a company right away?

Susan: I was an apprentice at Joffrey's, which at that time was allowing apprentices to perform with the New York City Opera. I danced that fall [1969] with the Opera. Then Joffrey II was formed and I was in that for a year and a half. I was 18 when I got into American Ballet Theatre.

Nancy: How did you get in?

Susan: The director of the Joffrey II, Jonathan Watts, helped me get into ABT classes to audition. I knew that Lucia Chase, the director of ABT, was watching me and I was waiting for her to say something about my joining the company but at that time Natalia Markarova had just come to New York and Lucia was always too busy to come and see the company's daily class. Finally after a month of taking class I was told that they wanted me to join the company.

Nancy: What kind of parts did you have at first?

Susan: Right away I danced in the corps of *Swan Lake*, *Giselle*, and *Copéllia*. Then in the next season I understudied a few soloist and demi-soloist roles. That summer I did the peasant girl in *Swan Lake*. That was three summers ago. I've been with the company two and a half years.

Nancy: You did a marvelous job of the street dancer in *Petrouchka* today. How long have you had that part?

Susan: Since last summer when the regular dancer was away ill for some time. Now she and I take turns dancing the part.

Nancy: Which other roles have you danced?

Susan: I did Lizzie Borden as a child in *Fall River Legend* [Agnes deMille] and a nice part in *Pillar of Fire*. I especially enjoyed doing the cowgirl in *Rodeo*, which I did for the first time last April in Milwaukee, Wisconsin.

Nancy: As a child, did you always dream of being a prima ballerina someday?

Susan: As a child I don't think I thought of dancing as a career, as a way of earning a living and all. I loved to dance and spent most of my time dancing but it wasn't until I was about 14 that I thought about making a career of dancing.

Nancy: How did your parents feel about your decision?

Susan: My parents have always been behind me. They were willing to go along with whatever I thought was best, which was good because that put the responsibility on my shoulders. But they have always helped me financially and supported me in other ways as well.

Nancy: Have you ever studied modern dance?

Susan: Yes, with Pola Narinska in Washington. She was such an inspiration. I can remember when José Limón came and performed in *The Traitor* at the Washington Cathedral. At that time I was thinking seriously about modern dance as a career. Part of my interest was because at that time I didn't have an easy facility for ballet. I was tempted to move over to modern dance instead. It seemed such a free aspect of dance.

Nancy: Do you mean by that that modern dancers don't have to have the technical ability that ballet dancers do?

Susan: No, I can't say that. A good modern dancer works just as hard as a ballet dancer, but the image of a ballet dancer is very precise. The lines have to be perfect, and everyone knows what those lines are. In modern dance, although the technique must be as well developed, the dancer has a more free range of lines and forms to develop.

Nancy: In your modern dance background, then, you were exposed to choreography very different from that of, say, *Swan Lake*. What is your feeling about the difference between *Swan Lake* and Tudor's *Pillar of Fire*?

Susan: I like *Swan Lake* very much. But sometimes it is painful, physically painful, to dance and stand in line; at least for me, because I am very short and I am one of the first ones onstage. There is a lot of standing around in a precise position for a long time. One doesn't have to use such artistic thought in corps de ballet work like *Swan Lake*. The formations are the most important thing in complementing the principal dancers and helping to create the proper atmosphere. In a Tudor ballet, on the other hand, there is not the use of the corps in the same way. You can't rely on pure beauty or technical excellence for success in a Tudor ballet. The atmosphere has to be just right and the timing must be in perfect tune with the atmosphere. It is a very special kind of feeling when you know you have performed *Pillar* well.

Nancy: Do you work personally with Tudor when you are preparing for performances of his works?

Susan: Yes, and it is an incredible experience. He has such a fine mind and understands movement in a kind of unique way. He can be very kind and enthusiastic when you are dancing the piece the way he wants it danced. And he can really needle you and show his temper when he is displeased. I consider it a privilege each time he criticizes me because I learn so much from it. So far I have never wanted to fight back. But I don't actually surrender to him, either. He seems to respect the dancer who listens to him and finally accomplishes what he wants without losing her own identity in the process.

Nancy: What are some technical differences between performing a Tudor work and a nineteenth century work?

Susan: The main difference is that in Tudor dances you can't let preparation show. There is no getting ready for a movement. Every movement must flow smoothly out of the one before it because a continuous statement is being made that preparation would fragment. You have to move with strength without having it come off as strength.

Nancy: Tell me about some particular rehearsal with him.

Susan: Well, just recently for the Tudor night I was rehearsing for the part of the child, Aganippe, in his revival of *Undertow.*

I had just finished reading some [Konstantin] Stanislavsky, incidentally, which had a real bearing on the way Tudor works. The problem was that I was supposed to be moving away from the transgressor, the main character, as if in mild fear and not understanding. Tudor kept saying that it wasn't right, that it looked like I was 12, not 7. So, I went back in my memory to times when I had observed young children about 7 years old playing and I realized that they have virtually no tension in their hands. When I did the movement again, I took the tension out of my hands and Tudor stood silent, looking at me. He didn't say anything and I was expecting him to dismiss me in disgust or something. Finally he said quietly, "That was better. Within the theatre and atmosphere, that would be right."

Nancy: Do all the dancers enjoy working with him?

Susan: Yes, and I think it is primarily because he makes the dancers use what they have even if they don't have an easy facility. Whatever their greatest ability is he gets it out of them. It is far more developing for an artist than just routinely doing the steps the choreographer asks for. Tudor cares about the development and growth of the dancers he works with.

Nancy: Going beyond Tudor to someone like Joffrey, for instance, who makes use of movement that is about as modern as you can get without taking off the toe shoes, to what extent is that kind of movement based on the classical form?

Susan: Those dancers use the classical training to build up strength. All those dancers are very, very strong technically. What they do is very difficult. But their use of the classical form is not to develop a dancer artistically. Working with Tudor and deMille one becomes aware of an artistic side to dance, which is not always present in ballets performed by the Joffrey company. They both have their value, but they make use of the historical, classical form in different ways.

Nancy: What do you think the role of artistry is in a dancer's performance?

Susan: I think that dancers should try always to balance the technical skill with their artistic abilities. And dances by Tudor, deMille, and Robbins generally emphasize this balance more than some of the ballets in Joffrey repertoire.

Nancy: Susan, as far as certain dancers getting to perform certain roles, how much resentment is there among the members of the company toward the choosing of principals for parts?

Susan: Well, I am sure there is some, although today it does not affect me. In a company of our stature the dancers who are chosen as principals are chosen because they are good and not because they have political pull, though I'm sure that may play its part concerning individuals. But when I find myself feeling sour because someone got a part I would like to have had, I just sit down and try to figure out why and usually I come up with enough good reasons to make me get back to work and stop sulking.

Nancy: What do you think of modern dance technique as a preparation for a dancer versus classical technique?

Susan: That's hard. I think all dancers should have both. They should understand what the other does. First of all, as children we in America are started way too young in ballet training. Modern dance training is much better for young

children than ballet because its muscular forms are not so
rigid. Most of the dancing schools in America are commercial and they are bad physically for children. Children
always are put on pointe too early. I'd say 9 years old is a
good age to start ballet.

For the mature dancer it is hard to say which kind of
training is the most beneficial. I really believe they should
have training in both.

Nancy: .How would you describe the difference between the intent
of *Swan Lake* and that of *Pillar?*

Susan: Well, because *Swan Lake* is a fairy story, it touches the
audience differently than *Pillar* does. *Pillar* touches more
humanly. It deals with predicaments that just about everyone goes through in some way. The reaction to *Swan Lake*
comes primarily from its perfection and beauty rather than
from its applicability to our lives. But both are important
ballets.

Nancy: What do you think of Alvin Ailey's work?

Susan: He has done work for the ABT and I have really enjoyed
the freedom of his movements. But the interesting thing
is that sometimes he tries to put his choreography on
pointe and it doesn't always work. His movement is so
different and often ballet-trained dancers can't do it. But
I enjoy it very much within his own company.

Nancy: Is it hard to dance to the music of many of Tudor's
ballets?

Susan: He's very subtle in the way he uses music. The dancers
have to be able to hear the same music Tudor is hearing.
And his musicality is very significant in the ballet. Sometimes it is very difficult to learn the music. [Arnold]
Schoenberg, for instance, is very difficult music. You have

to listen in an intense way. Sometimes you won't really hear it until you are doing it with an orchestra. You will rehearse over and over with the piano and then finally you rehearse with an orchestra and you suddenly hear the music he is talking about. *Undertow* is very hard to learn musically because it is a commissioned score. I don't like to count music, anyway. I prefer just to learn the music as music and not as counts.

Nancy: Who are your dance heroes or heroines from the past?

Susan: I like to read the historical accounts of the early first ballerinas like Taglioni and Pavlova. But I think even more than Pavlova I like reading about Olga Spessivtzeva. She was a ballerina from Russia born July 5th, 1895, who danced around Pavlova's time and she toured America, too. She was beautiful, very beautiful. Her *Giselle* was said to be one of the most touching ever seen. But she was not ever seen too much because in 1940 she became schizophrenic and she was put in a mental hospital until 1969. Now, interestingly enough, she is an old woman living in Nyack, N.Y., at the Tolstoy Foundation where Countess Tolstoy founded a home for refugee Russians. Helen Hayes is a friend of theirs. I saw a film of Spessivtzeva dancing and the blend, the balance of her technique and artistry was perfect. She wrote a book on technique for dancers and in it are technique exercises that are nearly impossible to do. She did them every day for years and years. It was amazing. She believed in studying movement from everyday life and real people, too. She studied people in an insane asylum before her performance of the mad scene in *Giselle*. Perhaps she got too involved. At one time she is said to have announced that she *was* Giselle. That was the beginning of her schizophrenia.

Nancy: You make a point of studying real people too, don't you?

Susan: Yes. If, for instance, I am supposed to dance as a little girl, my steps may be to walk, walk, relevé, piqué back, walk, walk, relevé, and so on. But I try to put into that structure something of the quality of a little girl walking on the cracks of a sidewalk or on the edge of a curb, the way children do. Dancing must be an expression of human feeling as much as possible. Within its forms, however strict, dancing must still be dancing.

BIBLIOGRAPHY

Amberg, George. *Ballet*. New York: Mentor Books, 1953. A good history of ballet beginning with Pavlova and going through musical comedy. Also includes summaries of the ballets.

Balanchine, George. *Balanchine's New Complete Stories of Great Ballets*. New York: Doubleday, 1968. Another excellent source for the stories of the great ballets. Also includes an essay on how to enjoy ballet and discussions of when young people should take lessons and a chronology of significant events in the ballet world.

Beaumont, Cyril W. *The Diaghilev in London*. London: Adam and Charles Black, 1951. A detailed account of this amazing man and his work. Practically a personal diary on the years Diaghilev spent in England.

————. *Three French Dancers*. London: Wyman & Sons, Ltd., 1934. Short, good biographies of Camargo, Salle, and Guimard.

Benois, Alexander. *Reminiscences of Russian Ballet*. London: Putnam, 1941. An invaluable insight into one of the most important times in the history of dance. Benois was stage designer with Diaghilev and has some interesting things to say about Fokine, Diaghilev, Nijinsky, and others. It also provides an insight into components of the ballet that are often overlooked.

Bourke, J. G. *Snake Dance of the Moqui*. Rio Grande. The first eyewitness of these sacred dances of the Hopi Indians tells with feeling and immense detail the fascinating story of this yearly rite. Important for broadening our view of the dance.

Buckle, Richard. *Nijinsky*. New York: Simon & Schuster, 1971. One of the finest biographies of a dancer ever written.

Brigham, John E. *The Graphic Works of M. C. Escher*. London: Oldbourne Book Co., 1967. This book does not purport to deal with dance but in fact it does, intimately so. Escher's works should be studied for their unparalleled dealing with movement.

Calvik, Romano. *Dance Year*. Boston: Dance Spotlight, 1964. A luscious collection of photographs of ballet, traditional and modern.

Chujoy, Anatole. *Dance Encyclopedia*. New York: A. S. Barnes and Co., 1949. A useful dictionary of dance if you are not looking for anything after 1949.

DeMille, Agnes. *Dance to the Piper*. New York: Bantam Books, 1953. DeMille is not only a first-rate choreographer and dancer but a writer as well. This autobiography is a treasure for anyone wanting to get an inside view of the hard road to the top.

————. *Lizzie Borden*. Boston: Little, Brown and Co., 1968. DeMille's zestful style tells the story of the making of one of her most famous dances, *Fall River Legend*. Before seeing this dance one should read this background.

————. *To a Young Dancer*. Boston: Little, Brown and Co., 1962. Another incomparable account of the dance world, this time directed specifically to anyone who takes dance seriously, as a career, that is.

Denby, Edwin. *Looking at the Dance*. New York: Pellegrini and Cudahy, 1949. A unique and fascinating collection of thoughts by one man on various aspects of dance. Reads like a diary and gives insights not found in other accounts of the dance. Particularly good because his comments were made at the time the dances premiered.

Fokine, Michel. *Memoirs of a Ballet Master*. Boston: Little, Brown and Co., 1961. A candid account of his successes. Excellent detail on his philosophy of dance. Also interesting as commentary on the relationships that formed this great period in dance history.

Goode, Gerald (Ed.). *The Book of Ballets.* New York: Crown Publishers, 1939. More summaries with 231 illustrations. Good on ballets choreographed before 1920. Nothing much after that.

Hall, Fernau. *The World of Ballet and Dance.* New York: The Hamlyn Publishing Co., 1970. A gorgeous photographic look at dance since Diaghilev. Text is brief but well written. A good way to begin a general education on the dance of the twentieth century.

Haskell, Arnold. *Ballet.* New York: Penguin Books, 1951. Haskell is probably the most prolific writer on the subject of ballet. If his style is dry, it at least is dependably accurate and complete. Excellent source for stories of and histories of ballet from the early sixteenth century.

————. *Baron Encore.* London: St. James's Place, 1952. Another luscious picture book of the ballet.

H'Doubler, Margaret N. *Dance: A Creative Art Experience.* Madison, Wisconsin: University of Wisconsin Press, 1968. Excellent reading on dance in the abstract covering such topics as "A Cultural Survey," "Education Through Dance," "Technique and Expression," "Form as Organic Unity."

Horst, Louis. *Modern Dance Forms in Relation to the Other Modern Arts.* San Francisco: Impulse Publications, 1961. A fine technical weaving of modern dance and such things as primitivism, medievalism, cerebralism, impressionism.

Humphrey, Doris. *The Art of Making Dances.* New York: Grove Press, 1959. The only book-length discussion of how modern dances should be created. Brilliant, easy to read, filled with the warm personality of one of the world's finest dancers.

Hunter, Sam. *Modern American Painting and Sculpture*. New York: Dell Publishing Co., 1959. Modern painting and modern dance have a lot to say about each other. This book should be part of any study of modern dance.

Hutchinson, Ann. *Labanotation*. New York: New Directions Books, 1954. A good basic study of the most widely accepted dance notation system.

Kahn, Albert E. *Days with Ulanova*. New York: Simon and Schuster, 1962. Kahn has photographed this world-famous ballerina as she is later in her life. It is an intimate acquaintance with a great woman. Photographs include Galina Ulanova as director, teacher, thinker, as well as dancer.

Kirstein, Lincoln. *Dance; a Short History of Classic Theatrical Dancing*. New York: Dance Horizons Inc., 1969. One of the best histories of dance. Weaves Kirstein's text with valuable quotations from major dance figures.

Kline, Peter and Nancy Meadors. *Physical Movement for the Theatre*. New York: Richards Rosen Press, 1971. An excellent guide to any study of movement. Contains exercises and suggestions for incorporating movement awareness into your life.

Kochno, Boris. *Diaghilev*. New York: Harper & Row, 1960. This book belongs on your coffee table with the Michelangelo and Leonardo art books. Beautifully compiled, fun to browse through. A general history of Diaghilev's years as promoter of the ballet.

Krokover, Rosalyn. *The New Borzoi Book of Ballets*. New York: Alfred A. Knopf, 1956. A detailed, well-written summary of all the best-known ballets and their creators. Told in narrative highlights.

Lawson, Joan. *A History of Ballet and Its Makers*. New York: Pitman Publishing Corporation, 1964. An excellent sketch of the history of ballet. Divided into sections that clarify the trends in dance since Greek days.

Leatherman, Leroy. *Martha Graham.* (Photographs by Martha Swope). London: Faber and Faber, 1967. An exquisite portrait of Martha with photographs of her dances since 1947 and of the revival of *Appalachian Spring* and *Cave of the Heart.* Text draws a moving picture of Martha at work.

Lloyd, Margaret. *The Borzoi Book of Modern Dance.* New York: Alfred A. Knopf, 1949. An indispensable guide to the history, personalities, and content of modern dance. Sensitively written with full chapters on all the major choreographers.

Martin, John. *The Modern Dance.* New York: A. S. Barnes and Co., 1933. A well-done discussion of the components of modern dance and its relation to beauty, art, intellectual perception, music, poetry, and other topics. To be acquainted with modern dance one must also be acquainted with John Martin.

Maynard, Olga. *The American Ballet.* Philadelphia: Macrae Smith Co., 1959. A more detailed look at a few of the important twentieth-century ballets and their choreographers. Covered are deMille, Lew Christensen, Eugene Loring, and Robbins. Includes also chapters on ballet schools and issues related to dance production.

McConnell, Jane T. *Famous Ballet Dancers.* New York: Vail-Ballou Press, Inc., 1944. A quickly moving account of fifteen dancers.

McDonagh, Don. *The Rise and Fall and Rise of Modern Dance.* New York: Mentor Books, 1970. A lucid account of the beginnings of modern dance and particularly of the more recent choreographers including Cunningham, Twyla Tharp, Meredith Monk, James Waring, Paul Taylor. The best source for discussion of current work in modern dance.

Meerloo, Joost. *The Dance—From Ritual to Rock and Roll, Ballet to Ballroom*. New York: Chilton Company, 1960. Title tells it all. Particularly interesting for nondance photographs that tie other kinds of movement into our notions about dance.

Morgan, Barbara. *Martha Graham*. New York: Duell, Sloan and Pearce, 1941. A priceless (and now out-of-print) companion to the Leatherman collection. Morgan's photographs cover Martha's dances up to 1940. These dances cannot be seen except through these photographs and the films in the New York Public Library for the Performing Arts.

Moore, Lillian. *Artists of the Dance*. New York: Dance Horizons Inc., 1938. Moore gives us biographies of the early dancers. Good on Taglioni, Fanny Elssler, and Noverre.

Nijinsky, Romola. *Nijinsky*. New York: Grosset and Dunlap, 1934. A completely personal view of the great dancer Nijinsky, written by his wife. Some interesting views of Diaghilev not usually found in more objective books.

———. ed. *The Diary of Vaslav Nyinsky*. Berkeley: University of California, 1971. Fascinating personal reflections of this fine artist.

Noverre, Jean Georges. *Letters on Dancing and Ballets*. New York: Dance Horizons Inc., 1966. (First publication 1801) An invaluable primary source on Noverre's famous revisions in dance.

Percival, John. *The World of Diaghilev*. London: Studio Vista Limited, 1971. This short book is as fascinating as the world it tells about. Pictures abound.

Puma, Fernando. *Seven Arts*. New York: Doubleday Inc., 1953. A must for placing dance in its rightful context with the other arts. Excellent article by José Limón. Also includes Frank Lloyd Wright, Aaron Copland, Thomas Mann, Leonardo da Vinci, Beethoven.

Reyna, Ferdinando. *A Concise History of Ballet*. New York: Grosset and Dunlap, 1964. A not so concise history that delivers a wonderful pre-twentieth century flavor of classical ballet.

Robert, Grace. *The Borzoi Book of Ballets.* New York: Alfred A. Knopf, 1947. Excellent brief summaries of the most famous ballets.

Ross, Nancy Wilson. *The Notebooks of Martha Graham.* New York: Harcourt Brace Janovich, 1973. A rare look at the actual mental and visual sketches Martha made before choreographing her masterpieces. Invaluable to anyone interested in the creative process.

Sachs, Curt. *World History of the Dance.* New York: W. W. Norton and Co., 1937. An excellent introduction to dance form of all kinds. Easy to read. Material is well sifted.

Seroff, Victor. *The Real Isadora.* New York: The Dial Press, 1971. Seroff gives us the life of Isadora without the sensational aspects that mar the truth in her autobiography. If you loved Isadora after reading her version of her life, you will adore her after seeing her through Seroff's supposedly more objective eyes.

Shawn, Ted. *Every Little Movement.* New York: Dance Horizons Inc., 1954. A book about François Delsarte and the application of his science to dance.

Sorell, Walter. *The Dance Has Many Faces.* New York: Columbia University Press, 1966. A marvelous collection of essays by the people who have made dance in America what it is. Includes essays by Humphrey, Limón, St. Denis, Frederick Ashton, Balanchine, Martin, Terry, Nikolais and many more. Reading the ideas of the choreographers themselves adds immeasurably to your understanding of the art.

Taper, Bernard. *Balanchine.* New York: Harper & Row, 1963. A close look at one of the most prolific and influential ballet choreographers in the world. Now in his fiftieth year of creating dances, Balanchine is still going strong. He is currently director of the New York City Ballet. Each year he turns out still more new work.

Terry, Walter. *Ballet.* New York: Dell Publishing Co., 1959. Brief summaries of the major ballets with a range of photographs up to modern pieces. Walter's style is delightful. He is an expert without the drag of expertise.

———. *Dance in America.* New York: Harper & Row, 1971. A sensitive summary of modern dance and ballet that America has produced. Some powerful photographs.

Tomkins, Calvin. *The Bride and the Bachelors.* New York: The Viking Press, 1968. A look at five masters of the avant garde, including Merce Cunningham. An excellent way to put modern dance in perspective with other very modern arts.

Wagenknecht, Edward. *Seven Daughters of the Theater.* Norman, Okla.: University of Oklahoma Press, 1964. An interesting combination of stars. In our attempts to make new relationships between ideas, it is fun to read a book that gives Marilyn Monroe equal time with Isadora Duncan.

Woody, Regina J. *Young Dancer's Career Book.* New York: E. P. Dutton and Co., 1958. Take a look at this if you are seriously considering dance as a career.

Zarina, Xenia. *Classic Dances of the Orient.* New York: W. W. Norton and Co., 1937. A good contrast and interesting context for our study of Western classical dancing.

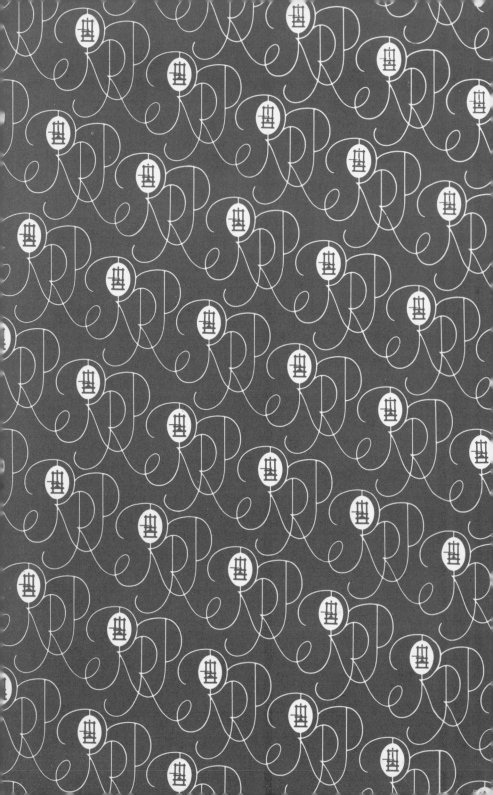